HEALTH CARE IN TRANSITION

PANDEMICS

EVOLUTIONARY ENGINEERING OF CONSCIOUSNESS AND HEALTH

HEALTH CARE IN TRANSITION

Additional books and e-books in this series can be found on Nova's website under the Series tab.

HEALTH CARE IN TRANSITION

PANDEMICS

EVOLUTIONARY ENGINEERING OF CONSCIOUSNESS AND HEALTH

PAVEL I. SIDOROV
EDITOR

nova
Medicine & Health
New York

Library of Congress Cataloging-in-Publication Data

ISBN: 978-1-53614-274-7

Published by Nova Science Publishers, Inc. † New York

CONTENTS

PREFACE

According to WHO, a pandemic is the spread of the disease on a global scale. The globalization of the modern world has led to a dynamic development of non-communicable epidemiology. That is why in this handbook we analyzed new etiopathogenesis mechanisms of clinical manifestations of classic and newest pandemics from influenza to mental illnesses. Particular attention is paid to integrative forms of care and early interventions based on the synergetic biopsychosociospiritual methodology of mental medicine. One can confidently say that at the maximum level of generalization, pandemics are instruments of civilizational management and evolutionary engineering of public health and consciousness.

Chapter 1. An infectious disease pandemic can have a significant effect on the human population with increased demand across the spectrum of health care from general practice for milder cases to intensive care for the most sick. Meeting the needs of people during a pandemic influenza shifts attention away from other areas of health care and increases waiting times in those other areas including for elective and other surgeries. The ability of a nation to respond to a pandemic depends on the extent of health resources, its disease surveillance capabilities, health system surge capacity, and access to health facilities.

During a pandemic absenteeism from work because of illness and fear of illness affects productivity and has an economic impact on the nation that can last for years. A nation's productivity, economy, trade capacity, defense, security tourism and other service industries are all vulnerable to the effects of a pandemic, especially if there is a second wave of infection.

The day-to-day lives of citizens would also be affected in other ways as measures are put in place to limit or contain the spread of the disease, such as social isolation, school closures, and travel restrictions. During a pandemic decisions will also be made regarding who will be treated when, and who will be left in avoidable pain and discomfort or possibly to die. This chapter will explore these and other non-health aspects of a pandemic drawing on past pandemics and relating those experiences to life in the twenty-first century.

Chapter 2. Influenza viruses affect most animals and can be transmitted to human sometimes causing pandemics. Many pandemics that have occurred in the last 100 years particularly that of 1918 and 2009 were caused by Influenza type A viruses of animal origin. Influenza A evolves frequently and unpredictably giving rise to novel strains, sometimes with enhanced transmissibility and pathogenicity in other animals and human. The 2009 H1N1 pandemic started in Mexico and was initially named 'swine flu' haven previously evolved in pigs undetected before it was transmitted to human. The virus also derived its gene constellation from avian, swine and human hosts. Since 1996, novel Highly Pathogenic Avian Influenza virus emerged from goose in Guangdong China and was transmitted to humans so far killing over 450 people worldwide. Similarly, a hitherto Low Pathogenic Avian Influenza H7N9 has already caused infection in 1557 people in China alone since 2013. Scientists are monitoring subtype H5, H7 and H9 of animal origin for influenza zoonoses and potentials to emerge as pandemic strain. This chapter reviewed the primordial, emerging roles and complexities of animal influenza viruses requiring critical assessments of the risks of human infection, prevention and management.

Chapter 3. Influenza pandemics have occurred four times in the past one hundred years, resulting in severe illness, hospitalizations and death amongst millions of people. Pandemics can also have serious socioeconomic consequences that disproportionately affect certain population groups. As there is likely to be little time between pandemic virus emergence and global transmission, effective and ethical pandemic preparedness is crucial.

The authors critically review the most recent Canadian and Ontario pandemic influenza plans, acknowledging that both are currently under revision. Using the principles of public health ethics and risk management, they assess potential avenues for improved pandemic preparedness. In particular, they consider the tensions and trade-offs between different ethical and risk management approaches. Drawing on a taxonomy of regulatory, economic, advisory, community and technological risk management options, the authors propose intervention strategies at the intersection of ethical and effective risk management practice.

Chapter 4. This chapter recommends using social media to automate the ability of organizations to coordinate their activities during pandemics. It is based on an innovative approach that constructs online networks of email and text messages as they evolve in real time. Based on a unique message addressing rule that takes advantage of "emergent intelligence", the approach shows how pandemics can be managed in real time. The author does this by tracking all communications in a chain of messages that are sent from person to person on a topic related to the pandemic. Then, as the community of interest grows, the approach creates a "closed network" that isolates it from the larger social network. The major benefit of this approach is that it provides feedback because it guarantees that all organizations in the network are automatically kept informed of all previous organizations that participated in the message chain. In this way, the author mimics the famous experiments of social psychologist Stanley Milgram, who provided the first empirical evidence of "six degrees of separation" when constructing paths via letters from person to person to achieve a goal.

Chapter 5. This is a study of suicides in the Russian Arctic with the focus on the Nenets Autonomous Okrug (NAO), a region with a large proportion of indigenous people.

As a starting point, the author conducted a retrospective population-based mortality study of suicides in the NAO, using data from the autopsy reports of suicide victims in the region in 2002-2012. Socio-demographic data were obtained from passports and medical records, and then linked to the total population data from the 2002 and 2010 censuses. Suicide rates for indigenous Nenets and non-indigenous population were calculated according to different socio-demographic characteristics, and corresponding relative risks for these two populations were compared. Variations in suicide methods, seasonal variations, and variations in the day of the week suicides occurred in the NAO were compared with national data from the Russian Federal Statistics Service (Rosstat). Forensic data on the blood alcohol content in suicide cases from the NAO were compared with the data from the neighboring Arkhangelsk Oblast.

Suicide rates in the NAO were higher than corresponding national figures. Suicide rates were higher among the indigenous Nenets than the non-indigenous population, and were associated with different socio-demographic characteristics. The author showed different relative frequencies of suicide by hanging, cutting, and firearm, as well as differences in suicide occurrence by month and day of the week in the NAO when compared with Russia as a whole. Alcohol may be an essential risk factor for suicide among the Arctic indigenous people.

The study results and conclusions may be useful to create suicide prevention programs that are targeted to different population groups in the Russian Arctic. The special emphasis should be done by the community based suicide prevention activities.

Chapter 6. The established feature of the modern world is a steady growth on the prevalence of all the major psychiatric disorders. The global predictor of this trend is the psychic traumatization of childhood and chronic psychosocial stress, triggering cumulative mechanisms of neuroepigenetic and epidemic development of mental immunodeficiency.

The task of the study is to describe the dynamics of the syndrome of mental immunodeficiency (SMID) in the early psychic traumatization of children. Mental immunity (MI) is a multimodal interface of consciousness and a biopsychosociospiritual identity matrix and the basis of security of the individual and society. The pathogenetic basis of the SMID is epigenetic accumulation in many generations of functional (reversible and dynamic) MI disorders that predetermine the change in the level and quality of mental health.

In the development of an epigenetic pandemic of traumatogenic mental immunodeficiency, six fractals are identified: 1) traumatogenic family; 2) pre-traumatic diathesis; 3) acute psychic trauma; 4) full-scale clinical picture; 5) chronization; 6) outcome. The main clinical manifestations of MI dysfunctions as a multimodal interface between identity and consciousness of an individual and habitat are described and systematized. Thus, the "missing link" between epigenetic pathogenesis and clinical pathoplasty of mental disorders is found. Multidisciplinary preventive-corrective and treatment-rehabilitation protocols and programs on the technological platform of mental medicine are proposed. The expression of Nobel laureate Peter Medawar, which became a textbook: "*Genetics* proposes, *epigenetics* disposes", is appropriate to be supplemented by the mission of mental medicine, which embodies and implements project models of quality and style, the image and meaning of life in the adaptive engineering and self-management of consciousness and health.

ACKNOWLEDGMENTS

The authors are sincerely grateful to the literary editor of the book, the scientific employee of the Institute of Mental Medicine of the Northern State Medical University – Maria Zaharova.

In: Pandemics
Editor: Pavel I. Sidorov
ISBN: 978-1-53614-274-7

Chapter 1

PANDEMICS: HEALTH AND OTHER RISKS

Rita Parker*[*], *PhD
Centre for European Studies,
Australian National University, Canberra, Australia

ABSTRACT

An infectious disease pandemic can have a significant effect on the human population with increased demand across the spectrum of health care from general practice for milder cases to intensive care for the most sick. Meeting the needs of people during a pandemic influenza shifts attention away from other areas of health care and increases waiting times in those other areas including for elective and other surgeries. The ability of a nation to respond to a pandemic depends on the extent of health resources, its disease surveillance capabilities, health system surge capacity, and access to health facilities.

During a pandemic, absenteeism from work because of illness and fear of illness affects productivity and has an economic impact on the nation that can last for years. A nation's productivity, economy, trade capacity, defense, security, tourism and other service industries are all

[*] Corresponding author: rita.parker@anu.edu.au.

vulnerable to the effects of a pandemic, especially if there is a second wave of infection.

The day-to-day lives of citizens would also be affected in other ways as measures are put in place to limit or contain the spread of the disease, such as social isolation, school closures, and travel restrictions. During a pandemic decisions will also be made regarding who will be treated when, and who will be left in avoidable pain and discomfort or possibly to die. This chapter will explore these and other non-health aspects of a pandemic drawing on past pandemics and relating those experiences to life in the twenty-first century.

Keywords: pandemic, resilience, systems perspective, societal functioning, non-pharmaceutical interventions, social distancing, absenteeism, economic impact, defense and security

INTRODUCTION

An infectious disease pandemic can have a significant effect on the human population with increased demand across the spectrum of health care from general practice for milder cases to intensive care for the most sick. Meeting the needs of people during a pandemic shifts attention away from other areas of health care and increases waiting times including for elective and other surgeries. The ability of a nation to respond to a pandemic depends on the extent of health resources, its disease surveillance capabilities, health system surge capacity, and access to health facilities.

While the health of a nation is affected by a pandemic, it also has a wider societal and economic impact. A nation's productivity, economy, trade capacity, defense, security, tourism and other service industries are all vulnerable to the effects of a pandemic. Pandemics cause enormous economic disruption and can quickly undermine communities and governance (Parker 2017). Responding to outbreaks once they have happened is far more expensive – in lives, money and other resources – than investing in preparedness. There is also an impact on human capital, the stock of knowledge and abilities in a population that contribute to a nation-state's productivity. The impact is even more significant when there is a second or even a third wave of infection. During a pandemic absenteeism from work because of illness, fear of illness, or caring for those affected also affects productivity and has an economic impact on a nation that can last for years.

In addition to the health effects, a pandemic can act as a stressor of a nation-state's social infrastructure, cohesion, prosperity and as a challenge to the machinery of government. The day-to-day lives of citizens is also affected in other ways when measures are put in place to limit or contain the spread of the disease, such as social distancing, school closures, and travel restrictions. This chapter will explore these and other non-health aspects of a pandemic drawing on past pandemics and relating those experiences to life in the twenty-first century. At the outset, the chapter sets out issues specific to a pandemic relating to lead-times and the availability of antivirals, personal protective equipment (PPE), and second and third waves of outbreak in a pandemic. The chapter then addresses several medical and health interventions, before focusing on non-pharmaceutical interventions and community mitigation. These issues set the context to examine the wider impact of a pandemic on civil-society and the implications for a nation-state and its future.

1. Methodology

The theoretical and methodological framework of research for this chapter enables analysis of a number of factors as they relate to each other, rather than adopting a narrower analytical approach. The issues have been considered within their broad contextual health and policy environments with the many different factors and actors that influence variables, and which may change at any time as part of an open system. A systems perspective assists in understanding the way these seemingly disparate issues are framed. This approach enables a holistic, strategic perspective, rather than a reductionist theoretical approach which focuses on separate components at the expense of other relevant variables. In this way, the wider aspects of civil-society affected by a pandemic can be understood in their totality.

2. Pandemic Setting

Pandemics are relatively rare events, but they have a significant effect on societal functioning. The World Health Organization (WHO) defines infectious diseases as caused by pathogenic microorganisms, such as bacteria, viruses, parasites or fungi; the diseases can be spread, directly or indirectly, from one person to another (World Health Organization 2017).

Pathogens, toxins and diseases are biological risks that can affect the well-being and security of a nation-state and its civil-society. In the inter-connected world of today, a localised epidemic can transform into a pandemic rapidly, with little time to prepare a public health response to halt the spread of illness. Previous pandemics have been variable in their impact but all have a common theme of destruction and mortality. Today, increased international travel, urbanisation, population growth, changing climate and weather patterns act as enablers that facilitate the spread of future pandemics. The World Health Organization has previously noted that the pandemics of the previous century encircled the globe in six to nine months, even when most travel was by ship. Given the speed and volume of international air travel today, viruses can spread more rapidly, possibly reaching all continents in less than three months.

An influenza pandemic occurs when two key factors converge: that is when an influenza virus emerges with the ability to cause sustained transmission from human to human, and there is very low, or no, immunity to the virus among most people. While most pandemics have been caused by various strains of the influenza virus, there have been some exceptions such as the Severe Acute Respiratory Syndrome (SARS) pandemic is 2003 and HIV/AIDS that continues to be a major global public health issue, having claimed more than 35 million lives so far. Globally in 2016, 1.0 million people died from HIV-related causes. There were approximately

36.7 million people living with HIV at the end of 2016 with 1.8 million people becoming newly infected in 2016 globally.

In an ideal situation, to address the health issues associated with a pandemic, a relevant vaccine is developed and delivered prior to the outbreak to prevent individuals from becoming sick with the virus and to achieve a certain level of saturation in order to protect the public. In reality, it takes months to develop a new vaccine after the first cases of outbreak appear and have been reported, noting that there is often a delay between when the first cases are presented and when they are reported and subsequently confirmed. During that time, the influenza spreads and, sometimes, the virus mutates thereby making it even more challenging to develop appropriate and effective vaccines. In situations where the influenza virus mutates as it replicates, these mutations can alter the virus enough so that older vaccines are no longer effective. While work is being undertaken to develop new vaccines, the virus continues to spread, and more people become ill, placing additional demands on medical and health services.

The demand on existing health and medical services and resources are often stretched beyond capacity during a pandemic. Results of a survey of the 2009 influenza pandemic (H1N1) impact on Australian emergency departments and their staff, showed a growth in demand and related emergency department congestion. These were highly significant factors causing distress within the departments (FitzGerald et al. 2010). Some survey respondents attributed the increased levels of stress and demand to media reporting. Presentation rates, particularly at clinics, are likely to be strongly driven by perception of the risk of infection. The type of media coverage can influence perceptions within communities about the severity of the virus. Too much media sensationalised reporting can imply that the spread is much worse than in reality and this increases uncertainty within a community. Alternatively, media reporting can present the impression that the infection rates of a pandemic are the same as, or less than, seasonal flu. In both instances, the media can influence perceptions and subsequent actions of members of the public. It can result in people who are well but fearful presenting at medical clinics or hospitals and thereby taking up valuable time and resources of medical staff. The imperative for health and other authorities is to ensure that timely, accurate and helpful information is available to members of the public.

Seasonal epidemics of influenza are different from a pandemic. For example, during the outbreak of H1N1 in 2009 it was initially perceived as a new virus, although death rates were similar or less than past seasonal influenzas. In 2009, generally younger people globally were more affected by the pandemic. This was reflected in those most frequently infected, and especially those experiencing severe or fatal illness. At the time, the most severe cases and deaths occurred in adults under the age of fifty years, with deaths in the elderly comparatively rare. This age distribution was in stark contrast with seasonal influenza where ninety percent (90%) of severe or fatal cases occurred in people sixty-five years of age or older (World Health Organization 2009).

Levels of preparedness for a pandemic vary around the globe and across the business and commercial sectors. The use of personal protective equipment - respirators, gowns, gloves, face shields, eye protection, and other equipment are necessary items for healthcare workers and others in their day-to-day patient care responsibilities. PPEs are also necessary for others who have daily contact with members of the public, such as in the service industries, public transportation sectors and emergency services. While the use of PPEs in a hospital or medical setting is generally considered to be the norm with an implied suggestion of assurance, their use in other settings can send a different type of message to the community – one of fear – if it is not accompanied by appropriate communication messages and information.

3. Second Wave Outbreaks

It is not unusual for there to be a second or even a third wave of outbreaks as part of a pandemic. During the 1918–19 pandemic three waves occurred. The initial first wave in the Spring and Summer of 1918 was relatively mild. It was followed by a severe and lethal second wave in the Autumn of 1918, and a subsequent third wave of less severity in the following season. The experiences of two other pandemics of the past century, in 1957 and 1968 revealed patterns of varying severity (Simonsen et al. 1998). Even if there is a pattern of mild illness, the impact of a pandemic during a second wave could worsen as large numbers of people become infected. Large numbers of severely ill patients requiring intensive care are likely to be the most urgent burden on health services, creating pressures that could overwhelm intensive care units and possibly disrupt the provision of care for people with other diseases and illnesses.

Gathering information year-round about influenza disease and viruses through the use of global and domestic disease and virologic surveillance systems are critical for the early identification of novel influenza A viruses that have pandemic potential. Monitoring of outbreaks from different parts of the world provides sufficient information to make some tentative conclusions about how an influenza pandemic might evolve. In 2009, the World Health Organization advised countries in the Northern hemisphere to prepare for a second wave of pandemic spread. It also advised countries with tropical climates, where the pandemic virus arrived later than elsewhere, of the need to prepare for an increasing number of cases (World Health Organization (2009a).

Between July 2009 to February 2011, Denmark experienced three waves of the pandemic influenza A (H1N1) in which two hundred and seventy-three patients were admitted to hospital. Patients hospitalised with pandemic influenza A (H1N1) were predominantly children and younger adults, and only a few patients were over sixty-five years of age. The third wave was the most severe when taking the number and percentage of patients admitted to intensive care units (ICU) and thirty-day mortality into consideration (Mølvadgaad 2013). This was noteworthy because the severity of hospitalised patients and requirement for ICU admission increased in the third (post-pandemic) wave compared to the second (pandemic) wave. This is in contrast to the reports from the 1918-19 influenza pandemic noted above (Barry et al. 2008).

New Zealand also experienced a second complete wave of pandemic influenza A(H1N1)2009 in 2010. Between April and December 2009, New

Zealand experienced the first wave of the influenza pandemic, with 3,211 laboratory-confirmed notifications, 1,122 hospitalisations and 48 deaths (Lopez & Huang 2010). The true extent of infection from the pandemic was much greater than indicated by surveillance data, with an estimated cumulative incidence of over 780,000 infections. This meant that the health of over eighteen percent (18.3%) of the population was affected directly by the pandemic. The second wave of the pandemic occurred in August 2010 and, although it was of similar duration to the first wave there were notable regional variations. By October 2010, there were 1,768 confirmed cases, including 732 hospitalisations and fifteen confirmed deaths (Bandaranayake et al. 2010). The figures, however, take no account of the wider societal, economic or personal impact on the population.

4. Medical and Health Interventions

Community-based medical and health interventions to reduce the spread and impact of pandemic influenza include immunisation and ongoing promotion of respiratory and hand hygiene. In some countries such as New Zealand, parallel interventions included the provision of free antiviral drugs. This was accompanied by requesting sick people to stay away from the workplace and from school, and to seek early medical advice.

Part of the range of medical and health policy interventions include isolation or quarantine, and treatment with influenza antiviral medications of all persons with confirmed or probable pandemic influenza. This presents particular strategic planning challenges for home-health, faith-based, and community organisations; medical providers; and public health agencies about how to coordinate care for those who would have to stay home because they are contagious or ill during a pandemic. There are particular additional challenges associated with caring for people who live alone. Notwithstanding the intended health benefits of medical and health interventions, a great deal of cooperation from the public is required to implement community mitigation measures successfully during a pandemic.

5. NON-PHARMACEUTICAL INTERVENTIONS

Communities play an important role in the prevention, early detection and early response to a pandemic. They can support the containment and control of infectious disease risks, limiting geographic spread and mitigating negative impacts by complying with the implementation of non-pharmaceutical interventions. The engagement of civil-societies during a pandemic to prevent, detect and respond to infectious disease risks is essential to ensure that efforts by governments are not delayed or negatively impacted. Communities form an integral part of a coordinated and collaborative effort between civil-society, the private sector and government. Such partnerships are most effective where there are established structures and systems in place, and preparedness plans are developed and built on trust that have been established before a crisis strikes (McClelland 2017).

In addition to medical and health interventions in the lead up to and during a pandemic, states can take a number of non-pharmaceutical actions in an attempt to limit the extent and reach of pandemics. Each action, however, has its own implications and consequences. Unfortunately, often a policy decision in one area is taken in isolation of the impact it will have in other areas. A policy of social distancing, for example, can have different implications depending on the extent it is applied or even enforced. Social distancing can include a range of stages along a spectrum. A policy of no physical contact such as shaking hands or embracing is relatively straightforward but it is difficult to enforce. Such a policy requires the cooperation of the wider community and it could have implications for other policy areas with associated legal and ethical considerations. For example, if stringent social distancing measures are put in place, police action may be deemed necessary if the situation is considered serious enough to warrant such levels of intervention.

Yet such responses challenge basic civil liberties and human rights. In 2006, the American Civil Liberties Union (Annas et al. 2006) was critical of the US Department of Health and Human Service's Pandemic Influenza Plan which posits a containment strategy that calls for massive uses of government force, for example to ban public gatherings, isolate symptomatic individuals, restrict the movement of individuals, or compel vaccination or treatment.

Other ethical issues arise as infectious diseases can highlight and deepen inequalities and vulnerabilities within civil-societies and accentuate existing disadvantages for some minority groups. Due to fear or ignorance, fringe groups such as the poor or disenfranchised could be discriminated against. In 1894, the City of Milwaukee in the United States responded to a smallpox epidemic by forcibly moving immigrants and poorer residents to a quarantine hospital (Walzer Leavitt 2003). The result was distrust and riot and the epidemic was not contained. Similarly, following the emergence of smallpox in Boston in 1902, police officers accompanied health officials to forcibly vaccinate immigrants and African Americans (Albert et al. 2001). More recently, when HIV first started to appear the only people being affected were described as the 'H-Group' that is, heroin users, homosexuals, and Haitians.

Different communities within multicultural societies such as Canada, the United States and Australia have specific needs during the planning and mitigation stages of a pandemic. In 2016, an Australian study was undertaken to develop an ethical framework to support implementation of an emergency response, with clear emphasis on planning with (not for) key populations, including Aboriginal and Torres Strait Islander peoples. The study outcome was to be used to focus on information acquisition and use, laboratory diagnostics, clinical trials, modelling and community engagement to contribute to Australia's emergency response to infectious diseases within a specific paradigm (McVernon et al. 2017).

The impact of the timing to implement and to cease interventions can also have unexpected effects on civil-society. In some instances, restrictions relaxed too soon have resulted in a re-emergence of infection requiring restrictions to be reintroduced, causing confusion, uncertainty and undermining the decision-making process and governance processes.

6. Social Distancing and Isolation

From a health perspective, an effective action that can assist in decreasing the rate of transmission of a virus is by reducing the social denseness of people in work, community, and school settings. During a pandemic, health and other authorities may wish to implement strategies to isolate or quarantine certain categories of people and, at the outset, it is important to clarify the distinction between isolation and quarantine. Isolation is the separation and/or restricted movement of people with a contagious disease from the larger population. Quarantine is a separation and restriction placed on the movement of people presumed to have been exposed to a contagious disease or suspected to be a carrier of a contagious disease. Isolation enables health authorities to conduct contact tracing from infected individuals and may result in the home quarantine of those exposed contacts. Quarantine measures enable health authorities to remove affected people from subsequent chains of transmission (Gostin et al. 2004). Ideally, from a health perspective, isolation and quarantine are most effective through the early detection of contagious disease cases and identification of possible carriers, however, isolation and quarantine actions require a delicate balance between the public good and individual liberties, with legal and ethical implications, as noted above. While voluntary isolation and quarantine are often successful, involuntary restriction may be deemed to be required in some circumstances or with particular individuals. Any plan for implementation of isolation or quarantine requires clear delineation of the relevant legal authorities and responsibilities. As such, it is imperative that public health personnel, law enforcement, the judicial system and other local authorities are familiar with these legal issues and that clear, accurate and timely information is made available to the general public.

With the developments in technology in the twenty-first century, it is possible for many people to work from home, however, this is not possible for workers in essential services such as hospitals, ambulances, fire, emergency services, and police and defense forces. While some degree of social isolation is possible, total isolation for the majority of the population is not feasible. Food and other provisions still need to be produced and bought or delivered to consumers. Online shopping and delivery is an area that is developing and could be utilised more during times of pandemic although it, too, is still vulnerable to absenteeism and is dependent on people being healthy, able and willing to work during a pandemic outbreak.

During a severe pandemic, public health authorities are likely to recommend that all, but the sickest people remain home while ill, with the most ill being hospitalised or in other care facilities. This strategy would have implications for large public gatherings such as sporting events, theatres, cinemas, political rallies or religious ceremonies or other mass gatherings of people that may need to be cancelled. In some cases, the organisers may not be able to recoup their out-of-pocket expenses and there may be an additional requirement to provide refunds if tickets have been sold. Issues may also arise if public transport services have been reduced or cancelled leaving groups of people stranded or unable to return home from large events if cancelled with little notice.

There are several practical concerns associated with implementation and enforcing a strategy of social distancing which would also have implications for the way people alter their working arrangements and schedules to decrease social density. The results of a national survey conducted in the United States to help public health officials understand the public's response to community mitigation interventions for a severe outbreak of pandemic influenza suggest that most respondents would comply with recommendations, but they would be challenged to do so if their income or job were severely compromised. During the 2003 Severe Acute Respiratory Syndrome (SARS) outbreak, public health officers in Toronto utilised voluntary quarantine and isolation measures to control its spread. Over 27,000 affected people were reportedly overwhelmingly cooperative with these requests. This high level of cooperation may reflect specific cultural traits of the Canadian population and cannot be extrapolated as a general indicator of compliance within other global civil-societies affected by an infectious disease pandemic.

The results also indicated that community mitigation measures could cause problems for people with lower incomes and for racial and ethnic minorities (Blendon et al. 2008). There are further implications and potential complications arising in situations when carers themselves become sick if they need to stay at home to care for an ill household member.

7. Voluntary Home Quarantine

An element of social distancing strategies to mitigate the spread of the pandemic is voluntary home quarantine together with the provision of antiviral medications as prophylaxis to members of households with confirmed or probable infection. This is dependent, however, on the availability of sufficient quantities of antiviral medications and a feasible means of distribution being in place. Voluntary home quarantine has implications for the individuals concerned regarding how they then access basics essentials such as food, medical care and medications. It can also affect the level and quality of productivity if people work from their home environment with the additional challenge of carers responsibilities, such as for young children or older members of the family, especially if those family members are contagious.

Isolation and quarantine measures raise a number of ethical principles that must be considered: the precautionary principle, use of the least restrictive alternative, a transparent public health system, a sense of fairness, just compensation for those impacted, keeping those subjected to isolation and quarantine in a humane environment, and abiding by the rule of law (Gostin et al. 2003). There is a fine balance between unnecessary quarantine and acting to limit the expose of individuals to a preventable disease, with subsequent morbidity and mortality. Each situation requires careful consideration.

8. School Closures

To minimise the spread of pandemic in a population the closure of schools and childcare facilities is an associated non-pharmaceutical intervention strategy to voluntary home quarantine. School closures take two forms, proactive school closure is when schools are closed before a pandemic reaches an area, whereas reactive school closure occurs because many students and staff are sick and the schools are not operating at the desired educational level.

If a decision is taken to close a school for health issues to limit transmission of the disease, consideration needs to be given to the range of other social and economic implications. In deciding to close schools, health and other officials must balance the potential health benefits of reducing transmission against high economic and social costs, ethical issues, and the possible disruption of key services such as health care, as well as the negative effects on households, the workforce, and the healthcare industry (Cauchemez et al. 2008). While older children could safely be left unsupervised at home, decisions to close schools also require strategies that prevent the re-congregation of children and teenagers in community settings. These issues present difficult challenges for authorities regarding how they might enforce such strategies. More vulnerable younger children would need to be cared for at home. This would require a working parent taking time off from their employment if other arrangements are not available. Taking time off work might be paid leave if it is available but in many instances such as for casual or part-time employees unpaid leave would be necessary.

The economic implications of a decision to close schools, even for a short time would not be insignificant. It is estimated that closing schools in the United States for an average of four weeks could cost up to $47 billion dollars (0.3% of GDP) and lead to a reduction of nineteen percent (19%) in key healthcare workers (Rutkowski 2010).

Home and distance schooling can assist students keep up with their curriculum. This is particularly critical in late high-school years when students are preparing for entry into tertiary education or to begin careers in the workforce. Failure to maintain educational progress can have longer term implications for the individual's earning capacity as well as the nation's overall productivity with longer term effects on its economy and potentially its defense and security.

9. Travel Limitations and Restrictions

The importance of public transport in a pandemic warrants attention as an enabler of the spread of infectious disease. Although some pandemic plans for transportation systems exist, these are often incorporated into all-hazards response plans. Most planning agencies focus on coordination of planning and actual response activities between different levels and types of organisations, and appreciate the importance of worker protection and vaccination, as well as effective distribution of vaccines and medical countermeasures. Nonetheless, often such plans do not address the specific requirements of people with access and functional needs, or address small urban and rural transit considerations. There are additional challenges when public transportation is limited due to absenteeism, and for smaller organisations that deal with the transportation of the elderly and disabled populations.

As a precautionary measure during a pandemic to complement other social distancing strategies, nation-states may put in place travel restrictions to and from their sovereign state as well as within it. While travel restrictions may slow the spread of infection, such measures do not stop the spread. After the emergence of the H1N1 influenza in 2009, some countries responded with travel-related controls during the early stage of the outbreak in an attempt to contain or slow down its international progress. These controls along with self-imposed travel limitations contributed to a decline of about forty percent (40%) in international air traffic to and from Mexico following the international alert. Nonetheless no containment was achieved by such restrictions and the virus was able to reach pandemic proportions in a short time (Bajardi et al. 2011).

In a review of twenty-three studies, there were initially positive outcomes with 'extensive travel restrictions' that limited more than ninety percent (90%) of movement. But those beneficial effects were erased when the transmissibility of the viral strain increased. Internal travel bans could delay pandemic spread by approximately one week, but international travel restrictions reduced pandemic attack rates by less than 0.02%. The review further found that at the local level, travel restrictions 'appeared to have limited effectiveness in the containment of influenza.' In Mongolia, for instance, a simulation restricting road and rail travel by ninety-five percent (95%) resulted in a 0.1% reduction in the pandemic attack rate. Similarly, in the United States, travel restrictions that were ninety-nine percent (99%) effective in barring entry of infected travellers resulted in a delay of pandemic spread by just two to three weeks. In the densely populated United Kingdom, a combination of internal and international travel restrictions might help to slow the effect of the pandemic within its borders but at the international level, travel restrictions had 'limited effectiveness,' with a forty percent (40%) restriction of air travel delaying by less than three days the advance of A(H1N1) from Mexico to other countries (Henderson 2014).

The issue of border control measures, including the possibility of border closures will impact many different categories of citizen, such as those in transit or foreign nationals from other nation-states. Those in transit may be prevented from continuing to another country. It is also possible that on return to their own country, they may be prevented from entering and, instead, be placed in enforced quarantine.

During a pandemic, decisions will also be made regarding who will be treated when, and who will be left in avoidable pain and discomfort or possibly to die. It also has implications for non-resident citizens and those in-transit from one country to another. Foreign nationals who might find themselves in a country with high levels of infection rates face other health and personal challenges. It is possible they may be placed in quarantine, or limited in the countries they are permitted for onward travel. Also, they might face the situation where no local assistance is available to them. This may be because the country they are in has limited or inadequate health resources and health system surge capacity. In other situations, it may be government policy not to provide assistance to foreign nationals.

At the time of the 2007 United Kingdom pandemic exercise 'Winter Willow,' there was a lack of clarity regarding what, if any, assistance would be offered to foreign nationals who may find themselves in the United Kingdom at the time of a pandemic. The UK policy at the time was that 'with the exception of emergency health care, no assistance will be offered to foreign nationals' with the intention of making that policy clear in future guidance (Department of Health 2007). There was no provision for the care of UK citizens abroad during a pandemic. This is in contrast to the French government's stated approach in its 2007 pandemic preparedness plan which makes provision under section eight for the management of French nationals abroad to be included as part of the Foreign Affairs Flu Pandemic plan which follows the WHO phases and states that it has scheduled the provision, as much as possible, of protection and healthcare means for all French nationals abroad, together with the intervention of a French resident doctor (or failing that, a local doctor) approved by the representational mission (General Secretariat for National Defense 2007).

10. Wider Impact of Pandemic on Society

10.1. Absenteeism

The World Health Organization has previously identified that a pandemic brings increased absenteeism in all sectors of the labor force, with capacity temporarily reduced in such essential public sectors as health care, law, enforcement, transportation, utilities, and telecommunications. In the 2007 United Kingdom pandemic exercise 'Winter Willow,' one of the lessons identified from the exercise was that business continuity would be a significant challenge for all organisations at all levels and during all stages of a pandemic, with absenteeism being a major obstacle to manage. It also identified a need for consistency regarding what services would and could continue to be delivered. A clear need was also identified for organisations to define more clearly their links to others, and to ensure their business continuity plans meshed with those of their partner organisations. Long periods of absenteeism also mean increased pressures and workloads for others in the organisation to address the inevitable back-log of work. This type of additional pressure can lead to an increase in accidents in the workplace. As such, organisations need to ensure their occupational health and safety procedures are adequate and implemented, and that there are good recovery plans in place.

The 2009 influenza A(H1N1) pandemic highlighted that while most businesses were aware of the need to be prepared, few had effective business continuity plans in place. A key concern was their limited ability to maintain operations successfully if a significant proportion of the workforce was absent due to the influenza outbreak. A 2008 study of the consequences of a severe pandemic in the United States found that thirty percent (30%) of all workers would become ill and 2.5% would die. Thirty percent (30%) of workers missing within a mean of three weeks of work would result in a decrease in the Gross Domestic Product of five percent (5%) (Jones et al. 2008).

In a further 2011 study based on the Centers for Disease Control and Prevention's FluWorkLoss program, using a thirty-five percent (35%) attack rate, a total of 47,270 workdays (or 3.4 percent of all available workdays) would be lost over the course of an eight-week pandemic among a population of 35,026 employees. The highest (peak) daily absenteeism estimate was 5.8 percent (minimum 4.8 percent; maximum 7.4 percent) (Thanner et al. 2011). Prophylactic absence from the workplace in response to fear of infection can add considerably to the economic impact of a pandemic and overall wellbeing of a civil-society. Decisions by individuals to take relatively drastic social distancing action to avoid infection increase rapidly over a short space of time and are likely to be influenced by the case fatality rate. This is supported by evidence from the public response to the H1N1 pandemic.

10.2. Economic Impact

Pandemic preparedness planning generally concentrates on population health and maintaining a functioning health sector with little focus on the wider economic and social impacts, with even less attention to ensure that economic risks of diseases are factored into macroeconomic assessments or to financial preparedness. Many lessons have been learned from past pandemics, yet a report in 2017 by the International Working Group (IWG) on Financing Pandemic Preparedness established by the World Bank, found that many countries are chronically under-invested in critical public health infrastructure. This includes facilities such as disease surveillance, diagnostic laboratories and emergency operations centres which are crucial assets in the early identification and containment of outbreaks, but which remain absent across several nations (The World Bank 2017).

The most obvious economic cost of an influenza pandemic is the cost of antivirals, immunisation drugs, medical staff and hospitalisation. But there are other less obvious but equally important economic costs for any nation-state during a pandemic and which often have implications for many months following.

When social distancing measures have been implemented, people stay away from work as well as public places such as shopping malls, cinemas and sporting events, tourist locations and other places with large groups of people. This results in a significant drop in consumer demand and consumption of goods and services. If a pandemic is ongoing for a long period, due to a second or third wave of outbreaks, it can negatively affect manufacturers and producers who cut output to align with lower demand. The result is a reduction to the number of workers engaged in these sectors, thereby reducing their overall, and disposable, income. If left unchecked, a negative spiral of economic and productivity decline can occur taking months or even years to recover.

During the 2003 SARS pandemic which lasted several months, international trade, travel, tourism, and migration flows were severely impeded and generated high levels of fear and psychological trauma in affected populations. China, Taiwan, and Singapore accounted for more than ninety percent of cases (Elbe 2009) and it had a significantly adverse effect on the Pacific Rim countries, most notably China and Canada. While the disease did not lead to the devastating health impact that many feared, there was a disproportionate economic impact (Smith 2006). According to the Asian Development Bank, SARS cost the Region between $18 billion to $60 billion in lost output (Fan 2003). Business and leisure travellers reduced their domestic and international air travel. The Park Place Entertainment which owns several gambling and hotel complexes in Las Vegas reported a fifty percent (50%) drop in net revenue attributed to the pandemic compared to the previous year. While at the same time Asia-Pacific airline carriers saw reduced revenue of $6 billion and North American airlines lost a further $1 billion (Begley 2013). Stock-market history shows that investors react to epidemics and pandemics but they also take into account other factors that may affect the movement of stocks and shares. In common with victims of the infectious diseases, market performance will also depend on the strength or weakness of prevailing conditions. For example, the avian flu pandemic of 1997 coincided with the Asian crisis, and preceded the Russian debt, and the Long Term Capital Management crises of 1998 which almost caused a global financial crisis.

A 2009 study estimated that the economic impact of costs related to pandemic illness on the United Kingdom would range from 0.5% and 1.0% of Gross Domestic Product (£8.4 billion to £16.8 billion) for low fatality scenarios. This estimate increased to 3.3% and 4.3% (£55.5 billion to £72.3 billion) for high fatality scenarios, and larger still for an extreme pandemic (Smith et al. 2009).

10.3. Tourism

Travel is an enabler of the spread of infectious diseases and the migration of humans has been responsible for disseminating infectious diseases throughout recorded history. The spread of the 1918-1919 influenza pandemic known as the Spanish flu followed the path of its human carriers, along trade routes and shipping lines (Billings 2005). Western Samoa lost twenty percent of its population and in India, which recorded up to fifty deaths per 1,000 people, up to sixteen million people died (Brown 1992). At the time of the Spanish influenza pandemic, nation-states imposed restrictions on public gatherings and travel. International travel today is now more extensive and far reaching. According to the World Tourism Organization, international tourist arrivals for 2014 exceeded 1138 million. Expansion in the global tourism market has contributed significantly to the spread of infectious diseases and human travel will continue to enable the emergence, frequency, and spread of infections in geographic areas and populations (McA Baker 2015).

While travel restrictions during a pandemic may have the effect of slowing the spread of the infectious disease, it also has an immediate and long term negative impact on the tourism industry which employs millions of people around the globe. Tourism is one of the fastest growing industries and is an important source of income for many countries including developing nations and those with limited or developing health services. The global tourism industry is also very sensitive to external events, such as a pandemic and it is deeply affected when international and domestic travel is restricted. The World Travel and Tourism Council estimated that approximately three million people in the tourism industry lost their jobs following the outbreak of SARS in China, Hong Kong, Vietnam and Singapore, resulting in losses of over 20 billion dollars in terms of GDP (Teitler-Regev et al. 2015). International tourism to Asia was badly affected by SARS, but the size of the effect varied with the destination country (McAleer et al. 2010).

10.4. Defense and National Security

Issues of national defense and security are not usually at the forefront of discussions about pandemics. Yet, it has been increasingly recognised that infectious disease can impact global security as well as that of individual nation-states. It has been argued that three viruses – HIV/AIDS, SARS and H5N1 – have 'done most over the past decade to place infectious disease issues firmly on the international security agenda' (Elbe 2011).

In July 2000 the landmark UN Security Council Resolution 1308 (United Nations Security Council 2000) declared HIV/AIDS a threat to international peace and security. This was the first time in the modern era that a public health issue was elevated to such status and it demonstrates a transformation in thinking about new risk and threats to security in the twenty-first century (Price-Smith 2009). The significance of the HIV/AIDS infection was again recognised in the context of defense and security in 2003 by then director of the Central Intelligence Agency (CIA) George Tenet when referring to HIV/AIDS stated that: "the national security dimension of the virus is plain ... it can undermine economic growth, exacerbate social tensions, diminish military preparedness, create huge social welfare costs, and further weaken already beleaguered states" (Tenet 2003).

During a pandemic the resources of a nation's defense forces would also be affected including the number of serving personnel available to support civil authorities. The types of defense support which would likely be in greatest demand during a flu pandemic include: providing disease surveillance and laboratory diagnostics; transporting response teams, vaccines, medical equipment, supplies, diagnostic devices, pharmaceuticals and blood products. It could also assist in treating patients, evacuating the ill and injured. It would also have a role in supporting law enforcement agencies controlling the movement into and out of areas, or across borders, with affected populations. The ability of the defense forces to provide support to civil authorities would be determined by the extent to which the pandemic had affected serving personnel, and other defense and security imperatives. This aspect is particularly pertinent to nation-states where there is civil or other conflict.

CONCLUSION

With random mutations that help them survive and adapt, new pathogenic microorganisms will inevitably find a way to break through existing health defenses and pandemics will recur in the future. Not only does a pandemic impose significant infrastructure demands on health care systems, but it exacts substantial economic costs in terms of sickness-related absenteeism from the workplace, schools and higher education institutions, and disrupted work schedules leading to lost productivity for civil-society. Such lost productivity can take months and even years to recover. Past pandemics have demonstrated the cost to the broader economy and to society as a whole associated with the non-health impact on civil-societies. This chapter has highlighted some of those issues. There are lessons from past pandemics for all nation-states and their civil-societies to prepare adequately for the next pandemic that could prove to be more devastating than previous ones if both health and the wider societal implications of a pandemic are not taken into account. In a pandemic the focus is on population health and the effective functioning of the health system, but wider consideration of the issues raised in this chapter is warranted for the overall well-being of civil-society and the security of nation-states.

REFERENCES

Albert, M. R., Ostheimer, K. O., Breman, J. G. (2001). 'The Last Smallpox Epidemic in Boston and the Vaccination Controversy, 1901-1903,' *New England Journal of Medicine*, pp. 344-375.

Annas, G. J., Mariner, W. K., Parmet, W. E. (2006). *Pandemic Preparedness: The Need for a Public Health – Not a Law Enforcement/National Security – Approach*, New York: American Civil Liberties Union.

Bajardi, P., Poletto, C., Ramasco, J. J., Tizzoni, M., Colizza, V. (2011). 'Human Mobility Networks, Travel Restrictions, and the Global Spread of 2009 H1N1 Pandemic,' *PLoS ONE* 6(1): e16591.

Bandaranayake, D., Huang, Q. S., Bissielo, A., Wood, T., Mackereth, G., Baker, M. G., et al. (2010). 'Risk Factors and Immunity in a Nationally Representative Population following the 2009 Influenza A(H1N1) Pandemic. *PLoS One*, Vol 5, Issue 100, e13211.

Barry, J. M., Viboud, C., Simonsen, L. (2008). 'Cross-protection between successive waves of the 1918–1919 influenza pandemic: epidemiological evidence from US Army Camps and from Britain.' *Journal of Infectious Diseases*, Vol 198, pp. 1427–1434.

Begley, S. (2013). 'Flu-conomics: the next pandemic could trigger global recession, *Reuters on line* at https://www.reuters.com/article/us-reutersmagazine-davos-flu-economy/flu-conomics-the-next-pandemic-could-trigger-global-recession-idUSBRE90K0F820130121.

Billings, M. (2005). *The Influenza Pandemic of 1918*, Stanford University, at http://virus.stanford.edu/uda/.

Blendon, R. J., Koonin, L. M., Benson, J. M., Cetron, M. S., Pollard, W. E., Mitchell, E. W., Weldon, K. J., Herrmann, M. J. (2008) 'Public response to community mitigation measures for pandemic influenza,' *Emerging Infectious Diseases*, Vol 14, Issue 5, pp. 778-786.

Brown, D. (1992). 'It All Started in Kansas,' *The Washington Post Weekly Edition*, 23-30 March 1992, Vol 9, Issue 21.

Cauchemez, S., Valleron, A. J., Boelle, P-Y., Flahault, A., Ferguson, N. (2008). 'Estimating the Impact of School Closure on Influenza Transmission from Sentinel Data,' *Nature*, Vol. 452: pp. 750-754.

Department of Health. (2007). *Exercise Winter Willow Lessons Identified*, UK Cabinet Office, at http://webarchive.nationalarchives.gov.uk/20080102111728/http://www.ukresilience.info/news/winter_willow_lessons.aspx.

Elbe, S. (2009). *Virus Alert: Security, Governmentality and the AIDS Pandemic*, Columbia University Press, Bognor Regis, West Sussex, England.

Elbe, S. (2011). 'Pandemics on the Radar Screen: Health Security, Infectious Disease and the Medicalisation of Insecurity,' *Political Studies*, Vol 59, Issue 44, pp. 848-866.

Fan, E. X. (2003). 'SARS: Economic Impacts and Implications,' *ERD Policy Brief No 15*, Asian Development Bank, Manila, Philippines.

FitzGerald, G. J. et al. (2010). *Pandemic (H1N1) 2009 Influenza Outbreak in Australia: Impact on Emergency Departments*, Queensland University of Technology.

General Secretariat for National Defense. (2007). *National plan for the prevention and control Influenza pandemic*, N° 40 /SGDN/PSE/PPS of January 9th 2007, Paris.

Gostin, L. O., et al. (2003). 'Ethical and Legal Challenges Posed by Severe Acute Respiratory Syndrome: Implications for the Control of Severe Infectious Disease Threats,' *Journal of the American Medical Association,* Vol 290, Issue 3229.

Gostin, L. O., Gravely, S. D., Shakman, S., Markel, H., Cetron, M. (2004). 'Quarantine: Voluntary or Not?' *The Journal of Law, Medicine & Ethics Special Supplement The Public's Health And The Law In The 21st Century,* pp. 83-86.

Henderson, D. (2014). 'Travel Restrictions Slow, but Do Not Stop, Pandemic,' *Medscape Medical News online* at https://www.medscape.com/viewarticle/835964.

Jones, D. A., Nozick, L. K., Turnquist, M. A., Sawaya, W. J. (2008). 'Pandemic Influenza, Worker Absenteeism and Impacts on Freight Transportation,' Hawaii International Conference on System Science, *Proceedings of the 41st Annual Conference*, 7-10 Jan. 2008, Waikoloa, HI, at http://ieeexplore.ieee.org/document/4438910/?reload=true.

Lopez, L., Huang, Q. S. (2010). 'Influenza in New Zealand in 2009' *Client report FW10019*. Upper Hutt: Institute of Environmental Science and Research; March 2010, at http://www.surv.esr.cri.nz/PDF_surveillance/Virology/FluAnnRpt/InfluenzaAnn2009.pdf.

McA Baker, D. (2015). 'Tourism and the Health Effects of Infectious Diseases: Are There Potential Risks for Tourists?.' *International Journal of Safety and Security in Tourism/Hospitality*, pp. 1-18.

McAleer, M. et al. (2010). 'An econometric analysis of SARS and Avian Flu on international tourist arrivals to Asia,' *Environmental Modeling and Software*, Vol. 25, No. 1, pp. 100-106.

McClelland, A. (2017). 'The Centrality of Communities and Civil Society in Epidemic and Pandemic Prevention. A Framework for Improved Preparedness and Response,' *Prehospital and Disaster Medicine Journal*, 32(S1):S205-S206.

McVernon, J., Sorrell, T. C., Firman, J., Murphy, B., Lewin, S. R. (2017). 'Is Australia prepared for the next pandemic?' *Medical Journal of Australia*, Vol 206, Issue 7, 17 April 2017.

Mølvadgaad, M., Linde Nielsen, H., Nielsen, H. (2013) 'The first, second and third wave of pandemic influenza A (H1N1)pdm09 in North Denmark Region 2009–2011: a population-based study of hospitalisations,' *Influenza and Other Respiratory Viruses*, Vol 7, Issue 5, pp. 776–782.

Parker, R. (2017). 'Pandemics and Dual-Use Research,' in Burke, A., & Parker, R., (Eds), *Global Insecurity*, Palgrave Macmillan, pp. 235-252.

Price-Smith, A. T. (2009). *Contagion and Chaos*, MIT Press, Cambridge, Massachusetts.

Rutkowski, M. J. (2010). *The Social and Economic Effects of School Closure During an H1n1 Influenza A Epidemic in the United States*, University of Pittsburgh at http://dscholarship.pitt.edu/6598/1/rutkowskimj_2010.pdf.

Simonsen, L., Clarke, M. J., Schonberger, L. B., Arden, N. H., Cox, N. J., Fukuda, K. (1998). 'Pandemic versus epidemic influenza mortality: a pattern of changing age distribution,' *Journal of Infectious Diseases*, Vol 178, pp. 53–60.

Smith, R. D. (2006). 'Responding to Global Infectious Disease Outbreaks: Lessons from SARS on the Role of Risk Perception, Communication and Management,' *Social Science and Medicine*, Vol 63, Issue 12, pp. 3113-3123.

Smith, R. D., Keogh-Brown, M. R., Barnett, T., Tait, J. (2009). 'The economy wide impact of pandemic influenza on the UK: a computable general equilibrium modelling experiment,' *British Medical Journal*, Issue 339, b4571.

Teitler-Regev, S. Shahrabani, S., Goziker, O. (2013). 'The Effect of Economic Crises, Epidemics and Terrorism on Tourism,' *International Journal of Business Tourism and Applied Sciences,* Vol. 1, No. 1, January – June 2013.

Tenet, G. J. (2003). *Testimony of Director of Central Intelligence, 11 February 2011,* Senate Select Committee on Intelligence, Washington DC.

Thanner, M. J., Links, J. M., Meltzer, M. I., Scheulen, J. J., Kelen, G. D. (2011). 'Understanding estimated worker absenteeism rates during an influenza pandemic,' *American Journal of Disaster Medicine,* Mar-Apr 2011, Vol 6, Issue 2, pp. 89-105.

The World Bank. (2017). *From panic and neglect to investing in health security: financing pandemic preparedness at a national level*, World Bank Group, Washington DC.

United Nations Security Council. (2000). *Resolution 1308 (2000): HIV/AIDS,* S/RES/1308 (2000), United Nations, New York.

Walzer Leavitt, J. (2003). 'Public Resistance or Cooperation: A Tale of Smallpox in Two Cities,' *Bioterrorism and Bioterrorism: Biodefense Strategy, Practice, and Science,* pp. 185-192.

World Health Organization, (2009), 'Global Alert and Response: Preparing for the second wave: lessons from current outbreaks' *Briefing Note #9*, World Health Organization, Geneva, (2009).

World Health Organization. (2009a). 'Preparing for the second wave: lessons from current outbreaks,' *Pandemic (H1N1) 2009* briefing note 9, 28 August 2009, Geneva, at http://www.who.int/csr/disease/swineflu/notes/h1n1_second_wave_20090828/en/committee on Intelligence, Washington DC.

World Health Organization. (2017). *Infectious Diseases Fact Sheet*, WHO Geneva.

BIOGRAPHICAL SKETCH

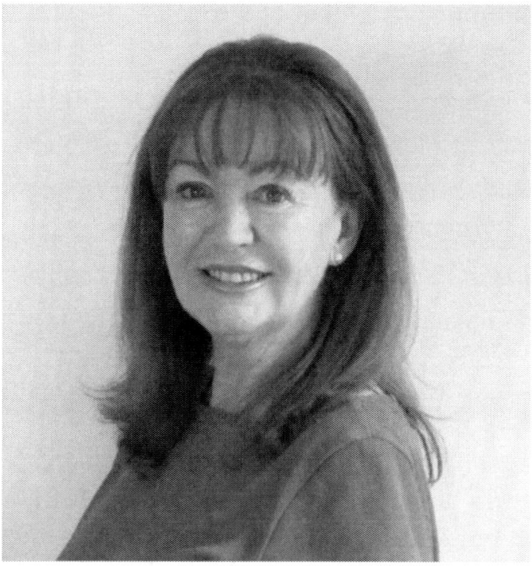

Dr Rita Parker is a Europa Visiting Fellow, at the Centre for European Studies, Australian National University and an Adjunct Associate Professor, University of Canberra (UC). She formerly managed the Australian Centre for Armed Conflict and Society, University of New South Wales (UNSW) at the Australian Defence Force Academy.

Prior appointments also include as Distinguished Fellow (Associate Professor) at George Mason University (GMU), Virginia, USA (2009-2014), Visiting Fellow UNSW Canberra (2011-2016). Dr Parker also held senior policy advisor roles in Australian Federal Government departments (including of the Prime Minster and Cabinet, Defence, and Attorney-General's) and to State governments, where she established her expertise in international transnational security and resilience issues. Among other areas Dr Parker's expertise was drawn on during the first Australian national pandemic exercise *Cumpston 06*, where she oversaw the national strategic arrangements across all jurisdictions. The outcomes from that Exercise informed future national response capabilities and strategies.

Dr Parker's current and ongoing research is focused on urgent global transnational security policy areas with a strong emphasis on actionable policy outcomes, within two thematic areas: non-traditional transnational security challenges to national resilience and, the future resilience of the liberal democratic model.

Dr Parker is co-editor of *Global Insecurity: Futures of Chaos and Governance* (2017). Her publications in 2018 include: *Unregulated population migration and other future drivers of instability in the South Pacific* (Lowy Institute, Sydney), and 'Pandemic: Health and other risks,' in *Pandemics: Evolutionary Engineering of Health and Consciousness* (Nova Science Publishers, New York).

Rita's research has been published in peer-reviewed journals and book chapters in Australia, Germany, Korea, Malaysia, Singapore and US, and she has been a regular columnist for *Security Solutions* magazine. Dr Parker's research takes an interdisciplinary approach and has been presented at national and international conferences.

Dr Rita Parker convenes Executive Education courses at the Institute for Governance and Policy Analysis, UC, and formerly convened the Executive Education course 'National Security Challenges and Policies in the Indo-Pacific,' at UNSW Canberra campus. She is a presenter for the UNSW Regional Security Issues course, and at the Australian Defence Force College on Europe's Contemporary and Future Challenges.

Dr Parker's contribution has been sought in high level policy forums. In April 2018 she was invited as part of the Australian delegation to participate in the EU-Australia Leadership Forum sectoral policy workshop on the rules-based international order in Brussels. Key recommendations from the workshop were subsequently presented to the official EU-Australia Strategic/Security Dialogue. In 2015 Dr Parker was invited to Berlin by the Konrad-Adenauer-Stiftung (KAS) to join the Australian delegation to take part in the high-level Dialogue Program with senior German Ministers and government officials in the lead up to the joint Ministerial meeting. While in Berlin she was also invited to present on the topic of unregulated migration and security at the KAS symposium with resulting follow up discussions and presentations with senior German officials.

Dr Parker was a founding Board member of the Australasian Security Professionals Registry (2011), and an invited member of the GMU Security Infrastructure Higher Education Initiative Speakers Bureau (2009). In 2016 she was invited to join the International Council of Security and Resilience Professionals. Dr Parker has advised organisations and corporations seeking to increase their corporate and organisational resilience and crisis management ability.

Education

- PhD – University of New South Wales, Canberra.
- Master of Business Administration, University of Canberra.
- Graduate Diploma, University of Canberra.
- Bachelor of Arts, Australian National University
- Security Risk Management Diploma, Canberra Institute of Technology

Professional Affiliations

- Member of the International Council of Security & Resilience Professionals
- Founding Board Member of the Australasian Security Professionals Registry
- Member International Studies Association
- Member Women in International Security
- Member Contemporary European Studies Association of Australia
- Member Political Studies Association of Ireland.
- Regular columnist, *Security Solutions* magazine.

Community activities

- Past President (2014-2016) and Member (ongoing) Women's International Club Inc
- Former Board member: Radio 1 RPH
- Former Board Member: the Commonwealth Club
- Volunteer News Reader: Radio 1RPH

Publication Highlights

Parker, R. (2018). 'Pandemic: Health and other risks,' in *Pandemics: Evolutionary Engineering of Health and Consciousness* Nova Science Publishers, New York (awaiting publication).

Parker, R. (2018). *Unregulated population migration and other future drivers of instability in the South Pacific,* Lowy Institute, Sydney.

Parker, R. (2017).'The European Liberal Democratic Model: Does it have a future in the Asia Pacific?' *Asia-Pacific Journal of EU Studies*, Vol 15, No 1. pp. 1-13.

Burke, A. & Parker, R. (Eds) (2017). *Global Insecurity*, Palgrave Press, London including two book chapters: R. Parker 'Pandemics and Dual-Use Research' pp. 235-252; R. Parker and A. Burke 'The United Nations and Global Security' pp. 347-368.

Parker, R. (2015). 'Food a Non-traditional Challenge to Security' in B. Mascitelli & B O'Mahoney (Eds), *Good Food for All: Developing knowledge relationships between China and Australia*. pp. 146-172. Connor Court Publishing Pty Ltd, Ballarat.

Parker, R. (2015). 'Lessons on Resilience,' *NFG Policy Paper Series*, Freie Universität, Berlin, 11/2015:1-15 Mar 2015.

Parker, R. & Stewart, J. (2014). 'Energy and Food Security,' *Security Challenges*, Vol 10 Issue 1, pp. 51-64.

Parker, R. (2013). 'Transnational Security Threats and Non-Traditional Security Challenges,' *The Journal of Defence and Security*, Vol 3, No 2, pp. 130-138.

Parker, R. (2013). 'Security is the Absence of Insecurity,' in B. Douglas (Ed), *Placing Global Challenge on the Australian Election Agenda*, Australia21, Canberra, pp. 42-44.

Parker, R. et al. (2012). 'System-Resilience Perspectives on Sustainability and Equity in Australia,' *Negotiating Our Future: Living Scenarios for Australia to 2050*, in M. R. Raupach et al. (Eds), Australian Academy of Science, Canberra, pp. 54-92.

Parker, R. (2012). 'Resilience as a Policy Response to Non-traditional Security Threats,' in H. Yan (Ed), *Society, Humanity and History*, IACSIT Press, Singapore, Vol 4.

Parker, R. (2012). 'Use of Soft Power and Its Impact on Security, *Putrajaya Forum*, edited proceedings, Malaysian Institute of Defence and Security, pp. 782-87.

Parker, R. (2011). 'All Hazards Resilience: A Paradigm for the 21st Century,' *Defence S&T Technical Bulletin,* Vol 4, No 1, pp. 56-63.

Parker, R. (2010). 'Organisations – Their Role in Building Societal Resilience,' in A. McLellan & M. Elran (Eds), *Proceedings of the First International Symposium on Societal Resilience,* Homeland Security Studies and Analysis Institute, Washington DC, pp. 263-282.

In: Pandemics
Editor: Pavel I. Sidorov

ISBN: 978-1-53614-274-7

Chapter 2

THE ROLE OF ANIMAL INFLUENZA IN PANDEMICS

Clement Adebajo Meseko*, DVM, PhD
Regional Centre for Animal Influenza and Transboundary Diseases,
National Veterinary Research Institute, Vom, Nigeria

ABSTRACT

Influenza virus affects most animals and can be transmitted to human, which may thereby cause pandemic. Many pandemics that have occurred in the last 100 years particularly that of 1918 and 2009 were caused by Influenza type A viruses of animal origin. Influenza virus evolves frequently and unpredictably giving rise to novel strains, sometimes with enhanced transmissibility and pathogenicity in other animals and human. The 2009 H1N1 pandemic started in Mexico and was initially named 'swine flu' having previously evolved in pigs undetected before it was transmitted to human. The virus also derived its gene constellation from avian, swine and human hosts. Since 1996, novel Highly Pathogenic Avian Influenza virus subtypes H5Nx emerged from goose in Guangdong China and was transmitted to human so far killing over 450 people worldwide. Similarly, a hitherto Low Pathogenic Avian

* Corresponding author: cameseko@yahoo.com.

Influenza H7N9 had already caused infection in 1557 people in China alone since 2013. Scientists are monitoring subtype H5, H7 and H9 of animal origin for influenza zoonoses and potential to emerge as pandemic strain. This chapter reviewed the primordial, emerging roles and complexities of animal influenza viruses requiring critical assessments of the risks of human infection, prevention and management.

Keywords: influenza virus, animal reservoirs, emerging pandemic threats, One Health

INTRODUCTION

The abundance and diversity of species in the animal kingdom relate to varieties of susceptible hosts of numerous pathogens, and human being occupies only a niche in this complex cycle of infection. Phylogenetic trees that are often used in the description of evolution and molecular epidemiology of pathogens have shown that the origin of emerging infectious diseases such as HIV, Ebola and influenza are vested in animals. Infectious diseases like influenza are also sustained by the interaction of one or more networks of similarly susceptible hosts in the animal kingdom that are also intricately linked with the environment. The potential inter-species connection and transmission of diseases, their sustenance in nature have long been recognized (Keesing et al. 2006). Expanded host range and diversity thus increase maintenance of pathogens in nature because other susceptible animals may serve as alternate host for the propagation of influenza virus beyond the primary host. Hence, the ability of pathogens to infect a wide range of hosts has been described as a risk factor for disease emergence in human, domestic and wild animals (Taylor et al. 2001; Cleveland et al. 2001). Though pathogen transmission within species is assumed to be higher than between species (Rudolf and Antonovics 2005), but when primarily host population is reduced or culled as control measure during influenza epizootics for instance, alternate susceptible host like duck become an important maintenance host. Waterfowls and other animals in nature thus serve as persistent reservoir/source of influenza from which transmission events may frequently occur. Monitoring animal influenza is therefore important for effective disease control and preventing pandemics.

1. Animal Influenza as Progenitor of Zoonoses and Pandemic Influenza Viruses

Aquatic birds are the natural reservoir of all subtypes of avian influenza virus (Alexander 2000). These viruses frequently mutate and reassort genes and may evolve into a highly pathogenic strain that can be transmitted to other animals including human or initiate a pandemic. Humans who are pre-exposed to influenza infection are also pre-immune to similar strains owing to their original antigenic sin and pre-existing partially cross-reactive immune responses in the host population (Wikramaratna et al. 2013; Vatti et al. 2017). Hence anamnestic immunity in the population serves as preventive measure except in the young, the aged and immune- compromised persons. On the other hand, individual or herd immunity to influenza in production animal is short lived due in part to short generation interval between breeding and slaughter or the entire life span thereby presenting new population of immune naive groups. Upon infection, influenza virus circulates, reassorts or mutates resulting in antigenic drifts and antigenic shifts more profoundly in animals with multiplicity of strains. However, epidemic behaviour in human is such that each strain of influenza elicit long-term partially cross-protective immune responses in addition to strain-specific immunity to limit infection except divergent strains from animal sources were introduced (Wikramaratna et al. 2013). Animals may therefore serve as donor of novel strains and precursor of divergent and potentially pandemic virus. The intensification of livestock production and co-mingling of multiple species contribute to narrowing human-animal interface and increase rate of exposure thereby promoting intra and interspecies transmission of antigenically divergent strains.

Pathogen ‘spill over and spill back’ are terminologies used by Daszak et al. (2000) to describe the transmission of infectious agents from reservoir animal population to wildlife (spill-over) or an epizootic/pandemic outbreaks of infection from wildlife to populations of susceptible domestic animals or human (spill-back). This clearly shows the dynamic of infectious diseases, particularly influenza virus, that have multiple susceptible hosts and the threat it poses to exposed human population. According to Morse (1994), reservoir animals play important role in the emergence and transmission of pathogens to human by providing zoonotic pool from which hitherto unknown pathogens or novel variants may emerge. Influenza is a classic example, where pandemics in humans occur after periodic exchange of genes between viruses of wild and domestic birds (aquatic and terrestrial) with humans directly or through intermediate host such as pigs. Direct transmissions of avian influenza to humans have also been described through analyses of the genes and occurred with Goose/Guangdong/1/96 lineages of H5, others include H7N4, H7N9 and H9N2 (Subbarao et al. 1988; Gao et al. 2013).

The greatest influenza pandemic in history often described as the mother of all pandemics was suspected to have been transmitted from an unknown avian host to human in 1918, and curiously before then, there had been a devastating fowl plague caused by avian influenza (Taubenberger and Morens 2006). As at 1918, it was not known whether the human pandemic had links with animal host until later revealed retrospectively that influenza viruses detected in swine and avian were descendants of the 1918 strain. While human influenza virus may have originated primarily from animal reservoir, ‘reversal of zoonoses’ has been used to describe the phenomenon where the virus already established in human, spill-back to animal host where they may then persist (Nelson et al. 2015). This virus mutates, reassorts and evolves a strain that is divergent and to which the human population may be susceptible thus sustaining the cycles of transmission from aquatic to terrestrial animals and human (Figure 1).

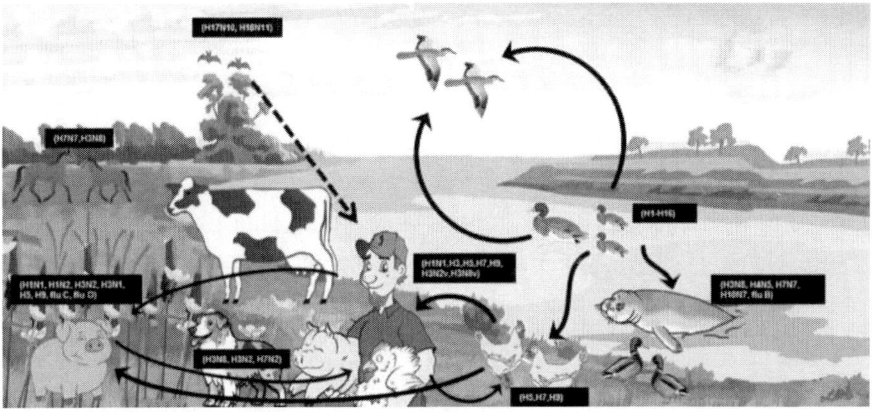

Figure 1. Illustration of aquatic and terrestrial influenza virus transmission cycles: infected migratory birds may introduce avian influenza virus across continents, domestic waterfowls in contact with terrestrial birds may be infected and transmit influenza virus to occupationally exposed persons, while interspecies transmission occurs in people, avian and other mammal.

To appreciate the role of animals in the emergence of influenza pandemics requires an understanding of the complexities of enzootic or epizootic influenza viruses when they emerge as genetically or antigenically novel in immunologically naive human. The virus is consequently able to cause infection with increase morbidity and or mortality as witnessed in 1918 and 2009 (Reid et al. 1999; Garten et al. 2009). It has been suggested that 1918 H1N1 pandemic was brought about by inter species infection from animal reservoir and gene adaptation in human. The hemagglutinins (HA) and neuraminidase (NA) surface proteins were derived from an avian-like influenza virus shortly before the beginning of the pandemic and the precursor virus had not circulated widely in human or swine in the years preceding outbreaks (Reid et al. 2000; Morens and Fauci 2007). The human population in that period were immune naive and that was suspected among other reasons why the 1918 pandemic was exceptionally severe (Taubenberger and Morens 2006). 'original antigenic sin' may confer strain specific or cross protective immunity on human, until a generation of naive hosts are born or molecular and biological adaptation in enzootic influenza virus in animal results in the emergence of a novel, immune evasive strain capable of successful infection that may be devastating.

The type of molecular and biological adaptation that can lead to emergence of novel virus is best envisaged in animal reservoirs and favourable conditions for subsequent interspecies transmission to human is often presented at the human-animal interface. This appeared to have manifested in 1997 in South East China, where the genes of isolates encoded the surface antigens (HA) and (NA) derived from the Goose/Guangdong/1/96 lineage with internal viral proteins from other sources including aquatic and terrestrial birds (Guan et al. 2002; Li et al. 2004). From 1997 through 2003 till present (2018), different genotypes of HPAI H5Nx have infected human and some lineage of the virus have already attained endemic status in poultry in Asia and some countries in Africa. The entrenched ecological niche of HPAI in poultry represents continuous pandemic threat to human through exposures in farms and live bird markets. Though according to Li et al. (2004) the H5 virus is yet to be efficiently transmitted from poultry to humans, and there is no conclusive evidence of sustained human-to-human transmission. However, continuous and extensive exposure of the human population to avian H5 viruses or other emerging subtypes H7 and H9 increase the likelihood that the viruses would acquire necessary molecular and biological features for efficient human-to-human transmission directly or via an intermediary like pigs.

Studies have established that aquatic birds are the primordial source of most influenza viruses in other animals including human (Hinshaw and Webster 1982; Webster et al. 1992). Animals therefore play a very important role in influenza epidemiology requiring constant monitoring as canvassed by the World Health Organization (WHO), Food and Agriculture Organization (FAO) and the World Organization for Animal Health (OIE) in the context of One Health. Scientists are encouraged to study influenza viruses in animals in order to understand the origin of zoonoses and pandemic influenza virus, and probably prevent global catastrophe (Morens and Fauci 2007; Mackenzie et al. 2013).

2. Natural Reservoir Host of Avian Influenza

The trajectory of evolution in the animal kingdom began in aquatic habitat. Aquatic birds are also the natural reservoir host of all H1 to H16 subtypes of avian influenza virus. These water birds, majority of which are in the order anseriforms (ducks, geese and swans) include about 180 species and charadriiforms also known as waders or shore birds (gulls, terns, plover, ibis) consisting of about 350 species, are recognized natural reservoir of influenza A viruses (Webster et al. 1992). Most waterfowls are wild and differ from domestic birds including poultry, though some of them have adapted to terrestrial habitat. Thus many wild birds are reservoir of avian influenza. Apart from waterfowls, other species of wild birds have also been infected by influenza virus including terrestrial and peri-domestic birds associated with agricultural areas (Morgan et al. 2015). Ducks are the most important reservoir of avian influenza among other waterfowls and play important role in the epidemiology serving as silent transmitter to other species, mammals and human (Olsen et al. 2006; Kim et al. 2009). H5N1 viruses have been isolated exclusively from waterfowls since 1996 and during 2000; however, from 2001 onwards they were isolated more frequently from both aquatic and terrestrial poultry, although the rate of non-symptomatic isolation remained the greatest in ducks (Li et al. 2004).

The concept of natural reservoir describes a host that may be infected but does not show symptoms of the disease and is therefore able to live with it and transmit the pathogen to other susceptible hosts. Haydon et al. (2002) defined reservoir as one or more epidemiologically connected populations or environment in which the pathogen can be permanently maintained and from which infection is transmitted to a target (susceptible) population. It was further elaborated that the existence of a reservoir is confirmed when infection within the target (susceptible) population cannot be sustained after all transmission between target and non-target (natural reservoir) populations has been eliminated. Hence, culling of poultry was expected to halt further transmission of avian influenza. However, the process did not eliminate the virus in its natural reservoir host as observed during slaughter of 1.5 million chickens in Hong Kong in 1998 and more culling in 2001 to prevent emergence of potential pandemic strain of influenza virus. The culling of domestic pigs in some countries to eradicate H1N1 in 2009 was also not able to stop transmission to susceptible individuals (Vogel et al. 1998; Meseko et al. 2013). This cycle or wave of transmission emanating from natural reservoir host to populations of susceptible host is often escalated by varieties of factors such as the ecology of natural reservoir host, human activities, alterations in the environment, weather and climate change. Since 2005, outbreaks of Goose/Guangdong/1/96 lineage H5 HPAI have occurred in waves across Asia, Europe, America and Africa closely associated with viral, host and environmental factors (Tassoni et al. 2015; Sims et al. 2017). The combination of these factors make outbreak forecasting more predictable and hence preparedness for disease outcomes, including management. However, the unpredictability of influenza virus in epizootics and panzootics is entrenched in natural reservoir host and the frequency of spill-over to domestic poultry and to cause human infections. The virus may probably be host and region localized/restricted and poses no immediate harm but intercontinental migration of wild waterfowls across continents results in global virus dissemination. The role of migratory waterfowls was less emphasised in the past until more recent revelations that migratory birds are important transmitter of avian influenza to new territories and playing a major role in the epidemiology of avian influenza globally (Cecchi et al., 2008; Tassoni et al. 2015; Sims et al. 2017).

The abundance of AI in waterfowls and as natural reservoir host also varies according to seasons from less than 10% in spring/summer to 10 - 60% in autumn/winter and during migration. This seasonal variation in prevalence is thought to be driven by the influx and aggregation of naive juvenile birds (amenable to infection) at breeding time and before or during migration, and may also be influenced by environmental conditions such as temperature and humidity, that can affect survival, hence persistence of virus in the environment (Olsen et al. 2006; Webster et al. 1992; Ellis et al. 2004). Typically the natural reservoir host that may be infected before migration could serve to transmit influenza virus across continents and to locations that were hitherto free of infection. The discreet habitat between aquatic species (waterfowls) and terrestrial birds (domestic poultry) means other intervening factors may play a bridging role in the transmission of AI from reservoir aquatic host to susceptible terrestrial species in farms/markets/environment and this may be ecological and anthropogenic in nature. Ecological factors like the presence of water bodies in wetlands where migratory or nomadic birds may stop, forage and winter have been identified as sources of infection for bridge species some of which are resident waterfowls, amphibious in nature and peri-domestic in habitat. Also speculated is the transmission of virus through shedding in feces, as waterfowls migrate across space, they contaminate environment accessible to feral birds. In an article published by Sturm-Ramirez et al. (2005) it was reported that there was a very strong association between HPAI outbreaks and the spatial distribution of ducks (domestic and free grazing) in Thailand, and the chronology of the different outbreaks across the country was an indication that ducks may have played a bridging role in the genesis of HPAI outbreaks among chickens (Gilbert and Slingenbergh 2004). Anthropogenic factor on the other hand involves such human activities like introducing potentially infected waterfowl from unknown sources to backyard poultry holding or offering potentially infected bird for sale in LBMs as is common in Asia and Africa (Meseko et al. 2007; Fusaro et al. 2009).

Apart from waterfowls serving as reservoir and transmitter of AI to domestic poultry, with potential for zoonotic spill over to human, persistence of AI in waterfowls also results in virus evolution and emergence in nature. Not necessarily evolutionary stasis (mutations in nucleotides that do not result in corresponding mutations in amino acid) as canvassed by Webster et al. (1992), where the virus appears to be fully adapted to its host and cause no overt clinical signs. The birds may also contribute to new infections or the endemicity of even the highly pathogenic influenza virus, where in many cases HPAI with multiple basic amino acid as determined by gene sequencing does not cause clinical sign or death but replicate efficiently in the host, and are readily transmitted to other susceptible hosts when in contact. Waterfowls therefore are sources of infection to other birds and create opportunities for expansion of its transmission to other species or silent circulation that enhances reassortment and mutations (Sturm-Ramirez et al. 2005; Meseko et al. 2007; Fusaro et al. 2009).

Aquatic birds provide all the gene pool of influenza A viruses (H1-H16) and genetically diverse strains that could reassort and emerge as pandemic influenza viruses for humans, lower animals, and other birds. Influenza virus adaptation from aquatic to its terrestrial host was suggested to be linked to the deletion in the NA stalk (Matrosovich et al. 1999). Beyond molecular features, it appears mixed poultry farming and rearing of waterfowls, like ducks, near poultry holdings, either in rural backyard farm or commercial holdings, appears to attract wild birds in search of food and water. Hence represent risks for transmission and establishment of AI in domestic poultry, humans and other mammals. Minimising contacts between poultry and waterfowls whether wild or domestic may therefore reduce the rate of viral spill over. In the same vein, safe human interaction with animals (wild, domestic and animal products) which includes adherence to biosecurity in farms, wildlife, fairs/markets may reduce zoonotic and pandemic influenza globally.

3. Diversity of Influenza Virus in Animals and Host Range

Apart from birds, other animals maintain influenza viruses in nature and these include swine, equine, canine, cattle, bats, whale and seal. Generally, there are recognised lineages of influenza virus according to species (avian influenza, swine influenza, equine influenza etc.) with an influenza virus from one host failing to replicate in another host (Ito and Kawaoka 2000). Infecting virus host range restriction factors have been ascribed to the HA, PB2 and NS1 proteins, particularly the binding preferences of the HA to host receptors and mutations in these protein plays an important role in overcoming the interspecies barrier and virulence in different host (Neumann and Kawaoka 2006). Interspecies transmission arises when for instance avian influenza virus adapted to other animals or humans by mutation or reassortment with circulating viruses in other species. The newly emerged or adapted viruses have the potential to cause pandemics in an immunologically naive human population (Cauldwell et al. 2014). An extraordinarily broad host range spectrum was observed for Gs/GD lineage of H5Nx that emerged in south East Asia affecting poultry, nearly all wild birds studied, and several mammals, including human were susceptible (Yamada et al. 2006). Avian influenza also has the propensity to mutate from LPAI to HPAI and the earliest record of HPAI occurred in wild birds that are typical reservoir host but succumbed to H5N3, infecting common terns (*Sterna hirundo*) in South Africa in 1961 (Becker et al. 1966). The different types of influenza virus in animals go through molecular and biological changes that allow virus to cross hosts species barriers.

The role of animals as a source of potentially hazardous influenza A viruses (from avian), arising through classical genetic reassortment or a novel adaptation to human receptors, necessitate monitoring of animals including swine for avian-like influenza viruses and should be integrated in Global Influenza Surveillance and Response System (GISRS) of the WHO and other international health plans or regulations (Ito and Kawaoka 2000).

While HPAI viruses can evolve directly from low-pathogenic (LP) virus precursors following introduction into domestic poultry and in avian species; infections with the H5 and H7 subtypes are of greatest concern because of their potential to evolve into the highly pathogenic form of the virus that can devastate poultry populations and occasionally be transmitted to humans (Monne et al. 2014). This underscores the need for a broad based surveillance and monitoring system of all animal influenza viruses as part of the strategy to prevent pandemics in human.

3.1. Avian Influenza

Most literatures describing origin of influenza virus in human often refer to the pandemic of 1918, and that outbreak in itself has also been linked with avian influenza. Unfortunately not many studies on avian influenza were documented until the 20th century and impetus to study avian influenza actually arose from observations on mammalian influenza virus (Alexander 2006). Though the clinico-pathological manifestation of avian influenza is very similar to that of an earlier known fowlpest also called Newcastle disease, an avian paramyxovirus recognized in 1926; but avian influenza virus is more related biologically to mammalian influenza virus and was thus classified alongside in the Orthomyxoviridae family (Kumar et al. 2018). Avian influenza however is different from other mammalian influenza in its host range and is widely distributed in aquatic birds: wild, free-living, captive and domestic. Influenza virus has been isolated from major families of birds including 105 wild bird species (Olsen et al. 2006). Waterfowls of the order Anseriformes and Chadriitoformes are by far predominant host of avian influenza where they are mostly asymptomatic existing as Low Pathogenic Avian Influenza (LPAI). It is only when LPAI mutates to the Highly Pathogenic (HP) variant which could cause severe mortality especially in domestic birds that it attracts attention. These mutations may be rapid after introduction from wild birds, sometimes it takes the LPAI virus to have circulated in poultry for a long period before mutation to HP takes place, hence unpredictable but the more the circulation of LPAI in poultry, the higher the chance that mutation to HPAI will occur (Alexander 2006). Mutation from LPAI and HPAI viruses resulting in outbreaks may also be as a result of a single introduction of LPAI virus with mutation to virulence occurring on a single influenza lineage, probably driven by evolutionary processes associated with the adaptation of the virus to a new host such as many times witnessed with waterfowl transmitting AIV to domestic poultry (Banjs et al. 2001). The classical case in point that has remained most severe and protracted in the recent past is H5NX from the Goose/Guangdong/1/96 lineage. The virus arose from reassortment in birds and different genotypes have circulated and evolved into various subtypes including H5N1, H5N2, H5N5, H5N6, and H5N8, some of which are more efficiently transmitted and cause disease in human. Many more avian influenza including H7N9 and H7N4 have also been transmitted from avian host directly to human and cannot be ruled out as potential pandemic strains requiring monitoring.

3.2. Swine Influenza

Swine influenza was not recognised until 1918 when pigs were also sickened by the prevailing influenza pandemic and the isolation of H1N1 virus from pigs in 1930 was the first biological identification of the causative agent of influenza. Shortly afterwards human influenza virus was also isolated and the epidemiological relatedness showed that these viruses were descendants of 1918 influenza pandemic (OIE 2009; CDC 2010). The swine H1N1 lineage that was acquired from human became enzootic in pigs for many years and was described as classical swine influenza virus, with the virus acquiring avian-like, human-like genes and triple reassortment events of avian, swine and human influenza in pigs (Ma et al. 2009). In 1976, influenza virus was apparently transmitted from closely quartered pigs to soldiers in a military base in New Jersey; the recruits consequently had influenza-like illness. The virus was identified as a strain of swine influenza known as A/New Jersey/76(Hsw/N1/swH1N1) (CDC 1997). Over the years close contact and co-mingling of animals promote intra- and interspecies transmission of diverse swine influenza strains from human and avian with the emergence of diverse subtypes including H1N1, H1N2, and H3N2 which are commonly detected. Reassortment between these subtypes, e.g., H1N1 and H3N2 resulted in another subtype H3N1 (Moreno et al. 2009). Enzootic swine influenza lineage circulates in different geographical regions (American, European and Asia) with some lineages dominating over the other and commonly detected in countries with swine influenza surveillance systems. In April 2009, a swine related influenza virus H1N1 caused another human pandemic which was also reintroduced in pigs in what has now been described as "reverse zoonoses". Apparently, humans can also transmit influenza viruses to pigs and zoonotic infections are not a one-way only event; they actually happen in both directions (Ma et al. 2009; Nelson et al. 2015).

The maintenance of influenza viruses in pigs and the frequent introduction of novel influenza viruses from other species contribute to the generation of strains of influenza virus with pandemic potential thus making pig a mixing vessel, and known to play important role in the epidemiology and evolution of new influenza viruses including pandemic strains (Ma et al. 2009). This trait in pig is enhanced due to the presence of both avian and human like receptors in their respiratory tract. This capability appeared to have manifested in the 2009 pandemic of H1N1pdm09 that originated in Mexico. The virus is a product of the combination of swine, avian and human influenza genes and must have circulated undetected in pigs until it eventually emerged in human in the form of a pandemic (Smith et al. 2009, Garten et al. 2009). It is becoming obvious from available records that the only time swine influenza virus attracts global public health attention is after pandemics in human. This happened in 1918 and 2009 following a period of circulation in human and eventual transmission to pigs. The strain thereafter became well established in swine where it could undergo some antigenic changes because of a lack of immune pressure unlike in human. Again, the influenza virus in pigs may resort with endemic swine, seasonal or pandemic human strains, to evolve another variant like the H3N2v already circulating in the United States (Wong et al. 2012). It is debatable if human may be a risk factor for pigs or vice versa in influenza epidemiology, but what is certain is the cyclical transmission of influenza virus between human and pigs which is important in the emergence and sustenance of an epidemic and this is more between human-pig-human than between any other species. Occasional transmission of zoonotic avian influenza from birds to human like the H5N1, H5N6, H7N9, and H9N2 has yet to acquire efficient human-to-human transmission and it is speculated that an intermediary host like the pig may make all the difference (WHO 2018).

3.3. Equine Influenza

Influenza in horses was suspected in 1299 and 1872, but like other influenza viruses that occurred before the advancement of science to precisely identify causative agents, most records are subjective (Xie et al. 2016). Most respiratory diseases often noticed in animals but of unknown etiology predate human influenza, but interestingly the disease often presents similar clinical manifestation in multiple species and appeared to have been transmitted from avian host to other mammals including horses in a spill over event that also may have caused illness in human (Morens and Taubenberger 2010). The first isolation of equine influenza virus (EIV) was in 1956 when subtype H7N7 was identified, and molecular evidence showed a relationship with avian influenza (Sovinova et al. 1958). The last isolation of this subtype was in the 1970s (Van Maanen et al. 2002). The second subtype of equine influenza (H3N8) remained enzootic in horses and has been transmitted to other animals including the dog, pig and cat (H3N8v) (Crawford et al. 2005, Tu et al. 2009). The H3N8 EIV appears to have emerged from an avian influenza virus that spread to horses (Murcia et al. 2011). Though serological Hemagglutinin tests (HI) have shown comparatively high affinity of horse red blood cells (RBCs) to avian virus, the evolutionary linkage is not fully explained (Odurinde et al. 2014). Horse RBCs also express a high proportion of SA α2,3-Gal linkages (avian-like receptors) compared with turkey RBCs and significantly improved sensitivity has been observed using horse RBCs for detecting HI antibodies to avian influenza H7N9 (WHO 2013). These are indications of biological relationship of equine influenza with avian hosts.

While equine influenza may not be typical fulminating zoonoses, there has been evidence of exposure in human who had close contact with horses and developed antibodies to the virus (Xie et al. 2016). Published records have shown some historical epidemics of human influenza that may have been caused by H3N8 EIV (Xie et al. 2016). In a report of one of the most devastating epizootic of equine influenza in Mongolia, 891,000 horses were affected with 176,000 deaths (about 20% case-fatality). Many persons who were occupationally exposed had influenza virus detected by molecular methods (Yondon et al. 2013). Similar exposures have also been reported in Australia and the United States clearly showing that human exposure and infection with equine influenza is possible with the possibility of interspecies mixes as horses still congregate with human in polo and horse racing events that could contribute to the epidemic of human influenza; however, the public health risk is as yet negligible (Meseko et al. 2016).

3.4. Canine and Feline Influenza

Two subtypes of canine influenza virus (CIV) have been identified in dogs viz: H3N8 and H3N2 and are characterized by fever, cough and pneumonia. H3N8 is an influenza virus strain transmitted from horses to dogs and was first identified in 2004 in racing dogs (greyhounds) in America. The infection was associated with pneumonia and extensive haemorrhages in the lung (Payungporn et al. 2008). Canine influenza subtype H3N8 is suspected to have jumped species from horses to dogs where it adapted to the new host through the accumulation of point mutations and has sustained dog-to-dog transmission (Buonavoglia 2007). Influenza H3N2 virus on the other hand was first identified in the United States in March 2015 following an outbreak of respiratory illness in dogs in the Chicago area and may be considered endemic due to continuous waves of outbreaks already in about 30 of the 50 States in America (Yin 2007). Prior to that, canine H3N2 influenza virus was restricted to South Korea, China and Thailand and likely transmitted from avian influenza viruses (H3N2, H5N1, H6N1, and H9N2) circulating in LBMs and poultry farms in Asia (Song et al. 2008). During the 2007 equine influenza outbreak in Australia, respiratory disease in dogs that were in close contact with infected horses was also observed and influenza (H3N8) virus infection was subsequently confirmed with genetic similarity to the infection in dogs (Kirkland et al. 2010). By 2018, canine influenza H3N2 has also been reported in Canada and was traced to importation of dogs from South Korea (Promed 2018); this strain was also transmitted to cats as it happened in 2016 and it may consequently adapt as another lineage of feline influenza.

Though severe illness due to influenza in cats has also been previously caused by H1N1pdm09 (Fiorentini et al. 2011). Recently, from December 2016 to February 2017, LPAI H7N2 subtype also caused illness in about 500 cats in the USA with signs of coughing, sneezing, and runny nose. Evidence of infection in one veterinarian who was involved in treatment of the animals was also recorded (Hatta et al. 2018).

As with most animal influenzas, cases of canine or feline influenza only become apparent when severe infection and or mortality is involved. Between 1984 and 2004, dog serum collected from racing greyhounds tested positive for canine influenza virus (CIV) and some positive tests were as far back as 1999 (Rosenthal 2007). What this shows is that infections with variants of influenza virus including H3N2 canine flu in human may also cause subclinical infection that is yet to be described and that co-infection of canine and human influenza may also result in reassortment that will become apparent when it causes illness given the close companionship that exist between human and dogs. It was similarly noted by Hatta et al. (2018) that close contacts between humans and their pets could lead to the transmission of feline viruses.

In an experimental study to understand infection dynamic in human and dogs, dog tracheas were inoculated with human influenza virus (HIV). Infected tracheal epithelium showed varied efficiencies and reassortant viruses carrying gene segments of CIV and HIV were viable. Addition of the hemagglutinin (HA) and neuraminidase (NA) of CIV to the 2009 human pandemic virus results in a virus that replicates at high levels and cause significant pathological lesions (Gonzalez et al. 2014). The authors concluded that there is a risk of anthropozoonosis and reassortment in dogs that might result in the generation of viruses carrying an H3 that is antigenically distinct from the H3 currently circulating in humans. This re-echoes the opinion of Song et al. (2008) whose virologic, serologic, pathologic, and phylogenetic analyses showed that cross-species infection of an entire avian influenza A virus (H3N2) in another mammalian species, raises the concern that dogs or cats may become a new source of transmission of novel influenza viruses.

3.5. Bat Influenza

Bats are mammal in the order *Chiroptera* but with fore limbs adapted as wings and are therefore the only mammal naturally capable of true and sustained flights like birds (Taylor 2005). Evolving arboreal habitat may have increased their capacity to harbour many pathogens including varieties of viruses without apparent clinical signs. According to Xie et al. (2018), bats can maintain just enough defences against illness without triggering a heightened immune reaction through dampened antiviral immune pathway called the STING-interferon pathway. Apart from lyssavirus, Ebola, Marburg, Hendra, Nipah, and SARS-CoV, Influenza A viruses quite different from other animal influenza have been detected in bats. Bats exist in large number, migrate and are interconnected and appear to maintain their own IAVs that are phylogenetically distinct and have not been detected so far in other mammals, hence their importance as reservoir is not yet known (Tong et al. 2012; Wu et al. 2014; Parrish et al. 2015). Nevertheless, influenza virus infecting any mammalian host is considered of greatest risk for zoonotic spread to human and the generation of pandemic or panzootics viruses (Tong et al. 2012). The bat influenza virus (bat/Guatemala/164/2009 (H17N10) discovered in Guatemala (Central America) has distant evolutionary divergence and was categorized as new subtype (HA17N10). It was also revealed that this lineage existed in nature as long as other animal influenza virus with which they share similar ancestors.

Similarly in Peru (Amazon rain forest region), another novel and distinct bat influenza A/bat/Peru/2010 (H18N11) was discovered and phylogenetic analyses between A/bat/Peru/10 and Guatemalan bat influenza viruses have shown more diversity. Bats may harbour more influenza virus genes than all other mammalian and avian species combined, indicative of a long-standing host-virus association (Tong et al.

2013). Interesting observation is that the bat virus evolved a different mechanism for virus attachment and release that is different from that which is conventional in influenza virus. The hemagglutinin and neuraminidase proteins showed that sialic acid is neither a receptor for virus attachment nor a substrate for release, suggesting a novel mechanism of influenza A virus attachment and activation of membrane fusion for entry into host cells. This is a new dimension: bats' potential as important reservoir for influenza viruses in human is yet to be fully unraveled (Tong et al. 2013).

Table 1. Distribution of influenza virus subtypes in commonly infected animals

Animal species	Influenza subtypes	Reservoir host or origin	Remark
Avian: *Anseriformes*- ducks, geese and swans *Chadriiformes*- gulls, terns, plover, ibis *Galiformes*- chicken, turkey, quail, guinea fowls	Hl to H16, N1 to N9 H5Nx, H7Nx,H9Nx	Avian	Natural reservoir host for most avian and mammalian influenza virus
Swine	H1N1, H1N2,H3N2, H1N3, H3N2v, H5,H9, flu C, flu D	Avian, human, Bovine	Mixing vessel for reassortment of diverse subtypes
Equine	H7N7, H3N8	Avian	Related to avian
Canine/feline	H7N8, H3N2	Avian, Equine	Spill over from horses and poultry
Bovine/Ovine/Caprine	Flu D	Not certain	Already described in many ruminants
Aquatic mammals: whale, seal	H1N1, H3N3, H3N8, H4N5, H4N6, H7N7 and H10N7, Influenza B	Waterfowls, human	Some sea mammals also act like mixing vessel
Bats	H17N10, H18N11	bats	Novel influenza A virus but highly divergent

An important observation on bat flu from zoonotic point of view is that it is compatible for genetic exchange with human influenza viruses in human cells, suggesting the potential capability for reassortment and contribution in the emergence of potential pandemic or panzootic influenza A viruses (Tong et al. 2012). This is particularly important when taken in the context of bats' abundance (1,200 species in the order *chiroptera*, representing over 20% of all mammalian species in nature) (Turmelle and Olival 2009), with global distribution across many social strata and dwellings amongst human in cities.

3.6. Bovine Influenza

Until April 2011, influenza virus classification in higher vertebrates included only genotypes A, B and C. Influenza D virus (D/swine/Oklahoma/1334/2011) originally detected in nasal swabs, collected from pigs exhibiting influenza-like illness in United States, has recently been characterized and is a new addition to the family *Orthomyxoviridae* (Hause et al. 2013). It is becoming a recurrent phenomenon with influenza genetic pool, that though the virus was first detected in pigs, it was discovered that the original host and reservoir is cattle. Hence the term bovine influenza is a more appropriate description as was later confirmed. In contrast to Influenza A with 8 RNA segments, influenza D virus has only seven RNA segments similar to influenza C but exhibits only approximately 50% overall amino acid identity to human influenza C virus and devoids of serological cross reactivity between the two (Wang et al. 2016). Influenza C has been previously detected in pigs in Beijing, China during 1981/82 but was related (though distantly) to human influenza C (Yuanji and Desselberger 1984; Hause et al. 2013).

Investigation of respiratory symptoms in swine and bovine herds in Italy also found influenza virus (D/swine/Italy/199723-3/2015) with genetic relatedness to the D/swine/Oklahoma/1334/2011 (Chiapponi et al. 2016). The same virus has also been identified in France and China, and found to replicate in ferrets, the animal model of choice for studying influenza virus susceptibility in human, suggesting that humans could be infected (Wang et al. 2016). The host range and geographic distribution needs to be further investigated though cattle have been suggested as the reservoir for this novel influenza virus (Hause et al. 2014; Ducatez et al. 2015). Considering that cattle is extensively kept as free range or in intensive ranches with increase chances of occupational exposure, more surveillance in other countries could reveal the extent of circulation of influenza D (bovine influenza) and its zoonotic implications.

3.7. Influenza in Aquatic Mammals

Although waterfowls and shore birds are aquatic in habitat, occurrence of influenza virus in birds have been previously discussed. Birds are however implicated in the transmission of influenza virus in aquatic environment to sea mammals (Hinshaw et al. 1984). The close antigenic and genetic relationship of influenza virus in aquatic birds and mammals is an indication that seabirds are source of infection. This is also more likely considering that influenza virus seeding and survival in high concentration in water by large congregation of water birds often in contact with other marine life. Influenza virus has been reportedly preserved in ice and water from high-latitude lakes that are visited by large numbers of migratory birds (Zhang et al. 2006). Many cases of IAV infection in marine mammals have also been documented with several IAV subtypes including H1N1, H3N3, H3N8, H4N5, H4N6, H7N7 and H10N7 most of which are transmitted from avian sources (Geraci et al. 1982; Hinshaw et al. 1984; Hussein et al. 2016).

Earlier record of influenza in aquatic mammal was the detection of the virus from whales (*Balaenoptera acutorostrata*) in the Pacific (Lvov et al. 1978). From 1979 to 1980, some harbour seals (*Phoca vitulina*) in Cape Cud, USA that exhibited respiratory signs and died in an unusually large numbers from pneumonia were sampled and tested for influenza virus. Influenza virus isolate, A/seal/Massachusetts/80 (H7N7) mostly identical to avian influenza strains was detected in the seals. Though all the genes are closely related to avian influenza viruses, biologically the virus behaves more like a mammalian strain, replicating in ferrets, cats, and pigs but not in avian species (Lang et al. 1981; Webster et al. 1981). This occurrence proved direct transmission and adaptation of influenza from avian species to sea mammals in the ocean. Further serological assays of the isolates showed that the H1 was more related to avian influenza and the N1 was related to equine source (H1avN1eq) demonstrating also that past and complex mixtures of gene pool and interspecies transmission was the origin of the virus that became adapted to the seal. Many years earlier in Russia, human influenza antibody had also been demonstrated in Pacific fur seal (*Caltvrhinus ursinws*), indicating a likely exposure at the human-animal interface (Sazanov et al. 1976).

In another event, influenza H3N8 virus, carrying mammalian adaptive mutations, was isolated from New England harbour seals in 2011 and the virus was found to have an avian-like receptor binding specificity, and could potentially establish infection in human lungs (Hussein et al. 2016). The outbreak was considered important because the virus naturally acquired mutations that are known to increase transmissibility and virulence in mammals. These include a D701N mutation in the viral PB2 protein, previously reported in highly pathogenic H5N1 avian influenza viruses infecting people. Seal was found to possess avian-preferred SAα-2, 3 and mammalian SAα-2, 6 receptors in their respiratory tract similar to what has been described in other mixing vessel like the pig (Anthony et al. 2012).

Influenza B virus was thought to be restricted to human until isolates (B/Seal/Netherlands/1/99) were recovered from a naturally infected harbour seal (*Phoca vitulina*) in 2012 and gray seals (*Halichoerus grypus*) were also found to be infected (Bodewes et al. 2013). Investigators suggested that influenza B virus infections can emerge in seal populations and that seals may constitute an animal reservoir from which human may be exposed to influenza B (Osterhaus et al. 2000). Seals are mammals like pigs and may play a similar role in the aquatic environment as pig does in the terrestrial habitat for the mixing of avian and human viruses (White 2013). Marine mammal populations with enhanced potential to infect humans could be a reservoir for adaptation of potentially pandemic human influenza virus. These cross-habitats and interspecies transmission of influenza virus show the need to also monitor spill over and adaptation of avian viruses in aquatic mammals to better understand zoonotic influenza that can contribute to emergence of pandemic strains from animal sources.

Conclusion: Emergence of Zoonotic and Pandemic Influenza Virus from Animals

Humans who are pre-exposed to influenza infection are immune to that strain or similar strains owing to the principle of original antigenic sin and its cross protection (Wikramaratna et al. 2013). Hence immunity due to anamnesis in individual host or population is a preventive measure against infection except in the young, the aged and immune-compromised. On the contrary, natural and passive immunity to influenza in animals is short lived due to short generation intervals when new populations of immune naive groups are born. Reassortments of influenza genes give rise to a new virus when two dissimilar IAVs infect the same host cell. The acquisition of viral gene segments from other sources in the course of persistent circulation in animals is a major risk factor. Repeated replication by error prone RNA also causes influenza virus to accumulate mutations to a level where it becomes antigenically divergent and unrecognized when transmitted to human even with pre-immunity. Sometimes escape variant in human may be due to immune selection pressure (Visher et al. 2016; Peacock et al. 2017).

In the 2009 pandemic, H1N1 influenza virus originating from animals was antigenically different from circulating seasonal H1N1 hence escaped immune recognition elicited by previously circulating seasonal H1N1 viruses and a pandemic ensued (Smith et al. 2009; Garten et al. 2009). While the mechanism for the emergence of novel influenza virus capable of initiating a pandemic may be intrinsic in the virus-host relationship, other factors relating to the host environment accelerate emergence of novel and pandemic virus from animals. These factors range from intensification of livestock production and co-mingling of multiple species (Sabir Bin Muzaffar et al. 2006; Gilbert et al. 2017). Hence interactions at the human-animal interface and ease of interspecies transmissions and spread of pathogens contribute to emergence of potentially pandemic influenza viruses from animals.

Once infected, influenza virus circulates more profoundly in animals with little immune pressure because animals are not routinely vaccinated against influenza virus. Animal influenza viruses that are precursors of influenza infection in humans are diverse and may be difficult to eradicate in nature, but the frequency of spill over transmission or interspecies transmission from animal sources can be drastically reduced. Measures that can reduce animal influenza virus introduction, circulation and adaptation in human would include monitoring and mitigating transmission cycles at the human-animal interface in the context of One Health. This is both economically desirable and a valid public health intervention for risk reduction, control and the prevention of a pandemic.

REFERENCES

Alexander, D. J. (2000). A review of avian influenza in different bird species. *Vet Microbiol*, 74:3–13.

Alexander, D. J. (2006). Avian influenza viruses and human health. *Dev. Biol* (Basel), 124:77–84.

Anthony, S. J., St. Leger, J. A., Pugliares, K., Ip, H. S., Chan, J. M., Carpenter, Z. W., et al. (2012). *Emergence of Fatal Avian Influenza in New England Harbor Seals.* mBio, 3: 4 e00166-12. doi: 10.1128/mBio.00166-12.

Banks, J., Speidel, E. S., Moore, E., Plowright, L., Piccirillo, A., Capua, I, et al. (2001). Changes in the haemagglutinin and the neuraminidase genes prior to the emergence of highly pathogenic H7N1 avian influenza viruses in Italy. *Arch Virol*, 146:963–73.

Becker,W. B. (1966). Isolation and classification of tern virus - influenza virus A/tern/South Africa-1961. *Journal of Hygiene-Cambridge*, 64(3): 309–320.

Bodewes, R., Morick, D., de Mutsert, G., Osinga, N., Bestebroer, T., van der Vliet, et al. (2013). Recurring Influenza B Virus Infections in Seals. *Emerging Infectious Diseases*, 19(3): 511–512.

Buonavoglia, C. and Martella, V. (2007). "Canine respiratory viruses". *Vet. Res*, 38 (2): 355–73.

Cauldwell, A. V., Long, J. S., Moncorgé, O. and Barclay, W. S. (2014). Viral determinants of influenza A virus host range. *J Gen Virol*, 95(6):1193-1210.

Cecchi, G., Ilemobade, A., Le Brun, Y., Hogerwerf, L. and Slingenbergh J. (2008). Agro-ecological features of the introduction and spread of the highly pathogenic avian influenza (HPAI) H5N1 in northern Nigeria. *Geospatial Health* 3(1): 7-16.

Center for Disease Control and prevention (CDC). (2010). *Key facts about swine influenza.* Retrieved from http://www.cdc.gov/flu/swine/key_facts.htm. (Accessed 23 March 2018).

Centers for Disease Control (CDC). (1997). Isolation of avian influenza A (H5N1) viruses from humans—Hong Kong. *MMWR* 46:1204-1207.

Chiapponi, C., Faccini, S., De Mattia, A., Baioni, L., Barbieri, I., Rosignoli, C. et al. (2016). Detection of Influenza D Virus among Swine and Cattle, Italy. *Emerging Infectious Diseases*, 22(2): 352–354. http://doi.org/10.3201/eid2202.151439.

Cleaveland, S. C., Laurenson, M. K. and Taylor, L. H. (2001). Diseases of humans and their domestic mammals; pathogen characteristics, host range and the risk of emergence. *Philos Trans R Soc Lond B Biol Sci.* 2001(356):991–999.

Crawford, P. C., Dubovi, E. J., Castleman, W. L., Stephenson, I., Gibbs, E. P. J., Chen, L. et al. (2005). Transmission of equine influenza virus to dogs. *Science.* 2005(310):482–485.

Daszak, P., Cunningham, A. A. and Hyatt, A. D. (2000). Emerging infectious diseases of wildlife: threats to biodiversity and human health. *Science*, 287: 443–449.

Ducatez, M. F., Pelletier, C., and Meyer, G. (2015). Influenza D Virus in Cattle, France, 2011–2014. *Emerging Infectious Diseases*, 21(2):368–371.

Ellis, T. M., Bousfield, R. B., Bissett, L. A., Luk, G. S., Tsim, S. T., Sturm-Ramirez, K. et al. (2002). Investigation of outbreaks of highly pathogenic H5N1 avian influenza in waterfowl and wild birds in Hong Kong in late 2002. *Avian Pathol*. 2004 (33):492–505.

Fiorentini, L., Taddei, R., Moreno, A., Gelmetti, D., Barbieri, I., De Marco, M.A, et al. (2011). Influenza A pandemic (H1N1) 2009 virus outbreak in a cat colony in Italy. *Zoonoses Public Health,* 58(8):573-581.

Fusaro, A., Joannis, T., Monne, I., Salviato, A., Yakubu, B., Meseko, C. et al. (2009). Introduction into Nigeria of a Distinct Genotype of Avian Influenza Virus (H5N1). *Emerging Infectious Diseases*, 15(3): 445–447.

Gao, R., Cao, B., Hu, Y., Feng, Z., Wang, D., Hu, W. et al. (2013). Human infection with a novel avian-origin influenza A (H7N9) virus. *N Engl J Med*, 368(20):1888-1897.

Garten, R. J., Davis, C. T., Russell, C. A., Shu, B., Lindstrom, S., Balish, A. et al. (2009). Antigenic and Genetic Characteristics of the Early Isolates of Swine-Origin 2009 A(H1N1) Influenza Viruses Circulating in Humans. *Science*, 325(5937):197–201.

Geraci, J. R., D. J., St Aubin, I. K, Barker, R. G., Webster, V. S., Hinshaw, W. J., Bean, H. L. et al. (1982). Mass mortality of harbor seals: pneumonia associated with influenza A virus. *Science*, 215 (4536):1129-1131.

Gilbert, M., and Slingenbergh, J. (2004). *Highly pathogenic avian influenza in Thailand: an analysis of the distribution of outbreaks in the 2nd wave, identification of risk factors, and prospects for real-time monitoring*. Food and Agriculture Organization of the United Nations and the Department of Livestock Development, Ministry of Agriculture and Cooperatives, Bangkok, Thailand.

Gilbert, M., Xiao, X., and Robinson, T. P. (2017). Intensifying poultry production systems and the emergence of avian influenza in China: a

"One Health/Ecohealth" epitome. *Archives of Public Health,* 75, 48. http://doi.org/10.1186/s13690-017-0218-4.

Gonzalez, G., Marshall, J. F., Morrell, J., Robb, D., McCauley, J. W., Perez, D. R. et al. (2014). Infection and Pathogenesis of Canine, Equine, and Human Influenza Viruses in Canine Tracheas. *J. Virol.* 88(16): 9208-9219.

Guan, Y., Peiris, J. S. M., Lipatov, A. S., Ellis, T. M. Dyrting, K. C. Krauss, S. et al. (2002). Emergence of multiple genotypes of H5N1 avian influenza viruses in Hong Kong SAR. *Proc. Natl Acad. Sci*. USA 99: 8950–8955.

Hatta, M., Zhong, G., Gao, Y., Nakajima, N., Fan, S., Chiba, S. et al. (2018). Characterization of a Feline Influenza A(H7N2) Virus. *Emerging Infectious Diseases*, 24(1), 75-86.

Hause, B. M., Collin, E. A., Liu, R., Huang, B., Sheng, Z., Lu, W., et al. (2014). Characterization of a novel influenza virus in cattle and swine: proposal for a new genus in the Orthomyxoviridae family. *MBio*, 5:2. e00031–14.

Hause, B. M., Ducatez, M., Collin, E. A., Ran, Z., Liu, R., Sheng, Z. et al. (2013). Isolation of a Novel Swine Influenza Virus from Oklahoma in 2011 Which Is Distantly Related to Human Influenza C Viruses. *PLoS Pathogens*, 9(2), e1003176.

Haydon, D., Taylor, L., Laurenson, K. Cleaveland, S. (2002). Identifying Reservoirs of Infection: A Conceptual and Practical Challenge. *Emerging Infectious Diseases*, 8(12), 1468–1473.

Hinshaw, V. S., and Webster, R. G. (1982). The natural history of influenza A viruses, pp. 79-104. In A. S. Beare (ed.), *Basic and applied influenza research.* CRC Press, Inc., Boca Raton, Fla.

Hinshaw, V. S., Bean, W. J., Webster, R. G., Rehg, J. E., Fiorelli, P., Early, G. et al. (1984). Are seals frequently infected with avian influenza viruses? *Journal of Virology*, 51(3), 863–865.

Hussein, I. T. M., Krammer, F., Ma, E., Estrin, M, Viswanathan, K., Stebbins, N. W. et al. (2016). New England harbor seal H3N8 influenza virus retains avian-like receptor specificity. *Scientific Reports*, 6: 21428. doi:10.1038/srep21428.

Ito, T. and Kawaoka, Y. (2000). Host-range barrier of influenza A viruses. *Veterinary Microbiology* 74: 71-75.

Keesing, F., Holt, R. D. and Ostfeld, R. S. (2006). Effects of species diversity on disease risk. *Ecology Letters*, 9: 485–498.

Kim, J., Negovetich, N. J., Forrest, H. L., and Webster, R. G. (2009). Ducks: The "Trojan Horses" of H5N1 influenza. *Influenza and Other Respiratory Viruses*, 3(4), 121–128.

Kirkland, P. D., Finlaison, D. S., Crispe, E., and Hurt, A. C. (2010). Influenza Virus Transmission from Horses to Dogs, Australia. *Emerging Infectious Diseases*, 16(4), 699–702.

Kumar, B., Asha, K., Khanna, M., Ronsard, L., Meseko, C. A., Sanicas, M. (2018) The emerging influenza virus threat: status and new prospects for its therapy and control. *Arch Virol.* 163(4):831-844.

Lang, G., Gagnon, A. and Geraci, J. R. (1981). Isolation of an influenza A virus from seals. *Archives of Virology* 68 (3-4): 189-195.

Li, K. S., Guan, Y., Wang, J., Smith, G. J., Xu, K. M., Duan L. et al. (2004). Genesis of a highly pathogenic and potentially pandemic H5N1 influenza virus in eastern Asia. *Nature,* 430(6996):209-213.

Lvov, D. K., Zdanov, V. M., Sazonov, A. A., Braude, N. A., Vladimirtceva, E. A., Agafonova, L. V. et al. (1978). Comparison of influenza viruses isolated from man and from whales. *Bull. Wld. Hlth. Org*. 56: 923—930.

Ma, W., Kahn, R. E., and Richt, J. A. (2009). The pig as a mixing vessel for influenza viruses: Human and veterinary implications. *Journal of Molecular and Genetic Medicine : An International Journal of Biomedical Research,* 3(1), 158–166.

Mackenzie, J. S., Jeggo, M., Daszak, P., Richt, J. A. (Eds.) (2013). One Health: The Human-Animal-Environment Interfaces in Emerging Infectious Diseases. In: *Current Topics in Microbiology and Immunology*. Springer Berlin Heidelberg.

Matrosovich, M., Zhou, N. N., Kawaoka, Y. and Webster, R. G. (1999). The surface glycoproteins of H5 influenza viruses isolated from humans, chickens, and wild aquatic birds have distinguishable properties. *J. Virol.* 73: 1146–1155.

Meseko, C. A, Oladokun, A. T. and Shehu, B. (2007). An Outbreak of Highly Pathogenic Avian Influenza (HPAI) In A Mixed Farm By The Introduction Of a Water Fowl. *Nigerian Veterinary Journal,* 28 (3): 67-69.

Meseko, C. A., Ehizibolo, D. O., Nwokike, E. C., and Wungak, Y. S. (2016). Serological evidence of equine influenza virus in horse stables in Kaduna, Nigeria. *Journal of Equine Science*, 27(3): 99–105.

Monne, I., Fusaro, A., Nelson, M. I., Bonfanti, L., Mulatti, P., Hughes, J. et al. (2014). Emergence of a Highly Pathogenic Avian Influenza Virus from a Low-Pathogenic Progenitor. *Journal of Virology*, 88(8), 4375–4388.

Moreno, A., Barbieri, I., Sozzi, E., Luppi, A., Lelli, D., Lombardi, G., et al. (2009). Novel swine influenza virus subtype H3N1 in Italy. *Veterinary Microbiology*, 138.3-4:361-367.

Morens, D. M. and Taubenberger, J. K. (2010). An avian outbreak associated with panzootic equine influenza in 1872: an early example of highly pathogenic avian influenza? *Influenza and Other Respiratory Viruses* 4(6): 373–377.

Morens, D. M. and Fauci, A. S. (2007). The 1918 Influenza Pandemic: Insights for the 21st Century. *The Journal of Infectious Diseases*, 195(7): 1018–1028.

Morse S. S. (1994). In: Emerging Viruses, S. S. Morse, Ed. (Oxford Univ. Press, New York, 1993), chap. 2; R. M. Krause, *J. Infect. Dis*. 170, 265.

Murcia, P. R., Wood, J. L. and Holmes, E. C. (2011). Genome-scale evolution and phylodynamics of equine H3N8 influenza A virus. *J Virol* 85:5312–5322.

Nelson, M. I., and Vincent, A. L. (2015). Reverse zoonosis of influenza to swine: new perspectives on the human-animal interface. *Trends Microbiol*, 23(3):142-53.

Neumann, G., and Kawaoka, Y. (2006). Host Range Restriction and Pathogenicity in the Context of Influenza Pandemic. *Emerging Infectious Diseases*, 12(6), 881–886.

Odurinde, O., Meseko, C. A, Ojalatan, J. D. and Oyeleye, A. F. (2014). Erythrocyte binding preferences and receptor specificities of influenza virus. 16th ICID Abstracts/*International Journal of Infectious Diseases* 21S: 1–460. DOI: https://doi.org/10.1016/j.ijid.2014.03.1338.

Olsen, B., Munster, V. J., Wallensten, A., Waldenström J, Osterhaus, A. D., Fouchier, R. A.(2006). Global patterns of influenza A virus in wild birds. *Science*, 312:384–388.

Osterhaus, A. D. M. E., Rimmelzwaan, G. F., Martina, B. E. R., Bestebroer, T. M. and Fouchier, R. A. M. (2000). Influenza B Virus in Seals. *Science*, 288(5468):1051-1053.

Parrish, C. R., Murcia, P. R., and Holmes, E. C. (2015). Influenza Virus Reservoirs and Intermediate Hosts: Dogs, Horses, and New Possibilities for Influenza Virus Exposure of Humans. *Journal of Virology*, 89(6), 2990–2994.

Payungporn, S., Crawford, P. C., Kouo, T. S., Chen, L., Pompey, J., Castleman W. L., et al. (2008). Influenza A virus (H3N8) in dogs with respiratory disease, Florida. *Emerg Infect Dis*, 14:902–908.

Peacock, T. P., Benton, D. J., James, J., Sadeyen, J.-R., Chang, P., Sealy, J. E. et al. (2017). Immune Escape Variants of H9N2 Influenza Viruses Containing Deletions at the Hemagglutinin Receptor Binding Site Retain Fitness In Vivo and Display Enhanced Zoonotic Characteristics. *Journal of Virology,* 91(14), e00218–17.

Promed (2018). *Influenza, Canine - Canada (02): H3N2, more canine cases.* Source: http://www.promedmail.org/post/20180115.5559485 (accessed 15-03-2018).

Reid, A. H., Fanning, T. G., Hultin, J. V. and Taubenberger, J. K. (1999). Origin and evolution of the 1918 "Spanish" influenza virus hemagglutinin gene. *Proc Natl Acad Sci U S A,* 96:1651–1656.

Reid, A. H., Fanning, T. G., Janczewski, T. A., Taubenberger, J. K. (2000). Characterization of the 1918 "Spanish" influenza virus neuraminidase gene. *Proc Natl Acad Sci U S A*; 97:6785–6790.

Rosenthal, Marie (July 2007). "CIV may have started circulating earlier than originally thought". *Veterinary Forum. Veterinary Learning Systems*. 24 (7): 12.

Rudolf, V. H. and Antonovics, J. (2005). Species coexistence and pathogens with frequency-dependent transmission. *Am. Nat.*, 166, 112–118.

Sabir Bin Muzaffar, Ydenberg, R., Jones, I. (2006). Avian Influenza: An Ecological and Evolutionary Perspective for Waterbird Scientists. *Waterbirds: The International Journal of Waterbird Biology*, 29(3), 243-257. Retrieved from http://www.jstor.org/stable/4132580.

Sazanov, A. A., Lvov, D. K., Btioude, N. A., Portyanko, V., Yaicova, S. S., Timofeeva, A. A., et al. (1976). Data on virological and serological examination of seabirds and fur seals in Tyuleryi Island of Sakhalinsk region. In: Lvov, D. K. (ed.), *Ecology of Viruses*. The D. I. Ivanovsky Institute of VirologT/, 4: 157-160.

Sims L., Harder, T. Brown, I., Gaidet, N., Belot,G., von Dobschuetz, S. et al. (2017). Highly pathogenic H5 avian influenza in 2016 and 2017 – observations and future perspectives. *FOCUS ON*, No. 11, Nov 2017. Rome.

Slusher, M. J., Wilcox, B. R., Lutrell, M. P., Poulson, R. L., Brown, J. D., Yabsley, M. J. et al. (2014). Are Passerine birds reservoirs for influenza a viruses? *J Wildl Dis*. 50(4):792-809.

Smith, G. J., Vijaykrishna, D., Bahl, J., Lycett, S. J., Worobey, M., Pybus, O. G. et al. (2009). Origins and evolutionary genomics of the 2009 swine-origin H1N1 influenza A epidemic. *Nature* 459:1122–1125.

Song, D., Kang, B., Lee, C., Saif, L. J., Ha, G., Kang, D. et al. (2008). Transmission of Avian Influenza Virus (H3N2) to Dogs. *Emerging Infectious Diseases*, 14(5):741-746. https://dx.doi.org/10.3201/eid1405.071471.

Sovinova O., Tumova B., Pouska F., Nemec J. (1958). Isolation of a virus causing respiratory disease in horses. *Acta Virol*; 2:52–61.

Sturm-Ramirez, K. M., Hulse-Post, D. J., Govorkova, E. A., Humberd, J., Seiler, P., Puthavathana, P. et al. (2005). Are Ducks Contributing to the Endemicity of Highly Pathogenic H5N1 Influenza Virus in Asia? *Journal of Virology*, 79(17): 11269–11279. http://doi.org/10.1128/JVI.79.17.11269-11279.

Subbarao K., Klimov, A., Katz, J., Regnery, H., Lim, W., Hall, H. et al. (1998). Characterization of an Avian Influenza A (H5N1) Virus Isolated from a Child with a Fatal Respiratory Illness. *Science* 279(5349): 393-396.

Tassoni, L., Fusaro, A., Milani, A., Lemey, P., Awuni, J. A., Sedor, V. B. et al. (2016). Genetically Different Highly Pathogenic Avian Influenza A(H5N1) Viruses in West Africa, 2015. *Emerging Infectious Diseases*, 22(12): 2132–2136. http://doi.org/10.3201/eid2212.160578.

Taubenberger, J. K. and Morens, D. M. (2006). 1918 Influenza: the Mother of All Pandemics. *Emerging Infectious Diseases*, 12(1): 15–22. http://doi.org/10.3201/eid1201.050979.

Taylor, L. H., Latham, S. M., Woolhouse, M. E. J. (2001). Risk factors for human disease emergence. *Philos Trans R Soc Lond B Biol Sci.* 356:983–989.

Taylor, P. (2005). Order Chiroptera/Bats. In J. Skinner & C. Chimimba (Authors), *The Mammals of the Southern African Sub-region* (pp. 256-357). Cambridge: Cambridge University Press. doi:10.1017/CBO9781107340992.018.

Tong, S., Li, Y., Rivailler, P., Conrardy, C.,Alvarez Castillo D.A., Chen, L-M., Recuenco, S. et al. (2012). A distinct lineage of influenza A virus from bats. *Proceedings of the National Academy of Sciences* Mar 2012, 109 (11) 4269-4274; DOI: 10.1073/pnas.1116200109.

Tong, S., Zhu, X., Li, Y., Shi, M., Zhang, J., Bourgeois, M. et al. (2013). New World Bats Harbor Diverse Influenza A Viruses. *PLoS Pathogens*, 9(10), e1003657. http://doi.org/10.1371/journal.ppat.1003657.

Tu J., Zhou H., Jiang T., Li C., Zhang A., Guo X. et al. (2009). Isolation and molecular characterization of equine H3N8 influenza viruses from pigs in china. *Arch. Virol.* 154:887–890. doi: 10.1007/s00705-009-0381-1.

Turmelle, A. S. and Olival, K. J. (2009). Correlates of viral richness in bats (order Chiroptera). *Ecohealth* 6: 522–539.

Van Maanen C. and Cullinane A. (2002). Equine influenza virus infections: An update. *Vet. Q.* 2002; 24:79–94. doi: 10.1080/01652176.2002.9695127.

Vatti, A, Monsalve, D. M., Pacheco, Y., Chang, C., Anaya, J. M., Gershwin, M. E. (2017). Original antigenic sin: A comprehensive review. *Journal of Autoimmunity,* 83: 12-21.

Visher, E., Whitefield, S. E., McCrone, J. T., Fitzsimmons, W., Lauring, A. S. (2016). The mutational robustness of influenza A virus. *PLoS Pathog* 12:e1005856. 10.1371/journal.ppat.1005856.

Vogel, G. (1998). Infectious disease: sequence offers clues to deadly flu. *Science.*279:324.

Wang, M., and Veit, M. (2016). Hemagglutinin-esterase-fusion (HEF) protein of influenza C virus. *Protein & Cell*, 7(1), 28–45. http://doi.org/10.1007/s13238-015-0193-x.

Webster, R. G., Bean, W. J., Gorman, O. T., Chambers, T. M., Kawaoka, Y. (1992). Evolution and ecology of influenza A viruses. *Microbiol Rev.* 56(1):152-79.

Webster, R. G., Geraci, J., Petursson, G., Skirnisson, K. (1981). Conjunctivitis in human beings caused by influenza A virus of seals. *N Engl J Med* 304, 911, 10.1056/NEJM198104093041515.

White, V. C. (2013). A review of influenza viruses in seals and the implications for public health. *US Army Med Dep J*, 45–50.

Wikramaratna, P. S., Sandeman, M., Recker, M., Gupta, S. (2013). The antigenic evolution of influenza: drift or thrift? *Philosophical Transactions of the Royal Society B: Biological Sciences*, 368(1614), 20120200. http://doi.org/10.1098/rstb.2012.0200.

World Health Organization (2013). *Serological detection of avian influenza A(H7N9) virus infections by modified horse red blood cells haemagglutination-inhibition assay.* WHO Collaborating Center for Reference and Research on Influenza. Chinese National Influenza Center. National Institute for Viral Disease Control and Prevention, China CDC. Source: http://www.who.int/influenza/gisrs_laboratory/cnic_serological_diagnosis_hai_a_h7n9_20131220.pdf. (accessed 8th March 2018).

World Health Organization (2018). *Influenza (Avian and other zoonotic) Fact sheet.* Reviewed January 2018. Source: http://www.who.int/mediacentre/factsheets/avian_influenza/en/ (accessed 8th March, 2018).

World Organization for Animal Health (2009). *Avian influenza, Scientific and Technical Review* 28. 1: 16-21.

Wong, K. K., Greenbaum A., Moll, M. E., Lando, J., Moore, E. L., Ganatra, R., et al. (2012). Outbreak of influenza A (H3N2) variant virus infection among attendees of an agricultural fair, Pennsylvania, USA, 2011. *Emerg Infect Dis*; 18(12):1937-44.

Wu, Y., Wu, Y., Tefsen, B., Shi, Y., Gao, G.F. (2014). Bat-derived influenza-like viruses H17N10 and H18N11. *Trends Microbiol* 22:183–191. 10.1016/j.tim.2014.01.010.

Xie, J., Li, Y., Shen,X., Goh, G., Zhu, Y., Cui, J., et al. (2018). Dampened STING-Dependent Interferon Activation in Bats. *Cell Host & Microbe*; 23(3):297–301.

Xie, T., Anderson, B. D., Daramragchaa, U., Chuluunbaatar, M., Gray, G. C. (2016). A Review of Evidence that Equine Influenza Viruses Are Zoonotic. *Pathogens,* 5(3). pii: E50. doi: 10.3390/pathogens5030050.

Yamada, S., Suzuki, Y., Suzuki, T., et al. (2006). Haemagglutinin mutations responsible for the binding of H5N1 influenza A viruses to human-type receptors. *Nature,* 444:378–382.

Yin, S. (2007). “Managing canine influenza virus”. *Veterinary Forum. Veterinary Learning Systems*. 24 (9): 40–41.

Yondon M., Heil, G. L., Burks, J. P., Zayat, B., Waltzek, T. B., Jamiyan B. O. et al. (2013). Isolation and characterization of H3N8 equine influenza a virus associated with the 2011 epizootic in Mongolia. *Influenza Other Respi. Viruses*, 7:659–665.

Yuanji, G., Desselberger, U. J. (1984). Genome Analysis of Influenza C Viruses Isolated in 1981/82 from Pigs in China: *Gen. Virol.* 65(11):1857-1872.

Zhang, G., Shoham, D., Gilichinsky, D., Davydov, S., Castello, J. D., Rogers, S. O. (2006). Evidence of Influenza A Virus RNA in Siberian Lake Ice. *Journal of Virology,* 80(24), 12229–12235.

BIOGRAPHICAL SKETCH

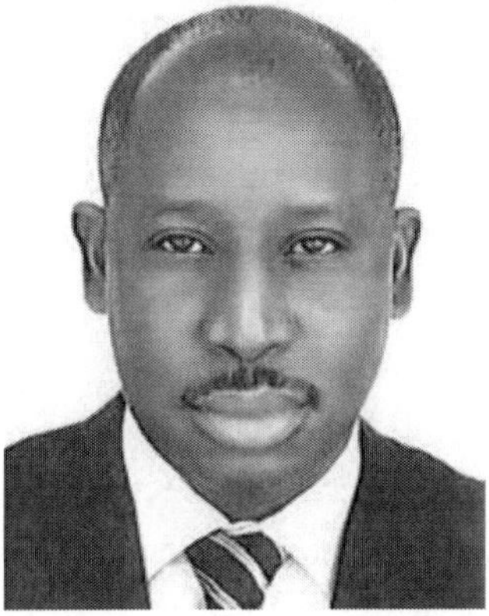

Clement Adebajo MESEKO; DVM, PhD. – Veterinarian/Virologist and infectious disease researcher, One health/Eco health advocate. Dr. Meseko is a Chief Vet Research Officer at the National Veterinary Research Institute, Vom, Nigeria. His research include influenza and other viruses of consequence with scientific ventures spanning field and laboratory investigation of causative pathogens of animal diseases, zoonoses, public and occupational health and at the human-animal-environment interface. To guide and optimize the impact of science on the society is an important aspect of his pursuit for positive research outcomes. He is currently a Research Fellow of the Alexander von Humboldt Foundation at Friedrich-Loeffler-Institut, Insel Riems, Germany.

As a Doctor of Veterinary Medicine (DVM) with a PhD degree in Virology, Dr. Meseko investigates infectious diseases including their diagnosis, research and control with focus on zoonoses; Influenza, Rabies, Ebola, Poxviruses, emerging and re-emerging pathogens and other transboundary animal diseases of economic/trade and health importance. With over 20 years combined professional working experience in many sectors of animal health and preventive medicine, his knowledge and areas of experience cover industrial-private sector, field activities in veterinary and human medical institutions/laboratories in many countries. Dr. Meseko has a good understanding of the dynamics of common diseases that threaten livelihood, global economy, and public health with published research outcomes in reputable journals. His present pre-occupation as a virologist comes with working within networks of international stakeholders in the industry, institutions, governments, NGOs and serving in technical groups and committees in many agencies including the FAO-OIE (OFFLU), WHO, IFPRI etc.

He is a trained and motivated professional with many years of multi- and inter-disciplinary experience in animal and human health laboratories at NVRI Nigeria (15 years), IZSVe Italy (1 year), NWHC Madison/ CDC Atlanta, USA, (3 months) and FLI in Germany (2 years). He has spoken in more than 40 national and international conferences and received more than 10 scientific awards for the promotion of his scientific ideals.

Upon graduation from Ahmadu Bello University in 1997, Dr. Meseko worked for five years in the private sector as Animal Health Technical Representative (Pfizer-Livestock Feeds PLC) and Territory Manager (Merial-Turner Wright LTD). Experiences accumulated over the years on myriads of animal diseases and the drive to unravel and proffer scientific solution motivated him to offer his service at the national and reference laboratory for veterinary research as Vet. Research Officer since 2002. His knowledge of influenza virology deepened in the course of training for Master's degree at the WHO National Influenza Centre (NIC) domiciled at the Virology Department, College of Medicine of the University of Ibadan. Research at the College of Medicine included providing laboratory support for patients with influenza-like and other respiratory infections at the Outpatient Clinic of the University Teaching Hospital, Ibadan. This period co-incided with the maiden outbreak of Highly Pathogenic Avian Influenza H5N1 in Nigeria in 2006 and sets the pace and place for his engagement on this pathogen of animal and human health implications in the last ten years.

His research activities manifested in various ways including OIE-FAO and World Bank assisted emergency control programmes for HPAI in Nigeria and pandemic preparedness of the WHO through which he attended many skill development trainings. Some of the research outcomes include the publication of 'Introduction into Nigeria of a distinct genotype of avian influenza virus (H5N1)' in *Emerging Infectious disease (EID)* in 2009 which chronicled genetic characterization of highly pathogenic avian influenza viruses (H5N1) isolated in Nigeria and revealed that a distinct genotype, never before detected in Africa, reached the continent. Phylogenetic analysis also showed that the viruses were genetically closely related to European and Middle Eastern influenza A (H5N1) isolated in 2007. Prior to that publication, Dr. Meseko and his colleagues in NVRI were able to demonstrate widespread activity of HPAI and published it in *Euro surveillance* as 'Serologic and Virological Surveillance of Avian Influenza in Nigeria, 2006-7'. Highly Pathogenic Avian Influenza devastated the poultry industry and threatens human health; the perceptions of risk among poultry workers were surveyed and published in EID in 2009. At this stage, Dr. Meseko intensified his passion for research in the course of his dual training in human and animal influenzas. To advance his professional knowledge and skill, he sought and obtained the World Bank; Robert S. McNamara (RSM) Fellowships for PhD research related to development. The award was implemented in both University of Ibadan, Ibadan and at the Istituto Zooprofilattico Sperimentale delle Venezia (IZSVe) in Italy. Painstaking scientific inquiry made possible by the grant award resulted in the detection of pandemic influenza subtype A/H1N1 in pigs for the first time in Nigeria and the second case in Africa showing evidence of reverse zoonoses as was also reported in other countries post the pandemic period. The result was published in *Veterinary Microbiology* in 2014 and a diagnostic autologous antigen/antisera was developed and produced for serological surveillance in Nigeria. During the time at the University of Ibadan, his knowledge of the ecology and dynamics of influenza virus was also demonstrated as supervisory assistant to postgraduate students of the College of Medicine. He participated in the design and execution of a Master's degree project that identified Low Pathogenic Avian Influenza (LPAI) H5N2 in domestic ducks at a live bird market in Ibadan. This was at a time when the country had been declared free of avian influenza. The outcome of this project was published in *Infectious disease of poverty* in 2014. The work monitored carrier hosts of avian influenza in Nigeria at a Live Bird Market (LBM) between July 2011 and July 2012. It described occurrence of LPAI in domestic ducks in Nigeria and underscored the importance of continuous surveillance and monitoring of influenza virus in order to prevent emergence of virulent strains that may spread to commercial poultry and infect humans.

The important role of private sector insight and multi-level partnership collaboration for surveillance and to achieve early detection/control of HPAI was proven when after about 10 years of disease free status, HPAI was re-introduced to Nigeria and West Africa. The identification of the index cases was through observations by a private Veterinarian in Lagos in consultation with Dr. Meseko's team at the regional laboratory in Vom. A diagnosis of new clade 2.3.2.1c was also made in partnership with OIE/FAO reference laboratory in Padova, Italy leveraging on established relationship. The event was reported in EID as 'Highly pathogenic avian influenza A (H5N1) virus in poultry, Nigeria, 2015. In the letter to the editor at Centre for Disease Control and Prevention (CDC), it was highlighted that: In Nigeria, from February 2006 through July 2008, outbreaks of highly pathogenic avian influenza (HPAI) subtype H5N1 virus infection in poultry negatively affected animal and public health as well as the agricultural sector and trade. These outbreaks were caused by viruses belonging to genetic clades 2.2 and 2.2.1. In January 2015, seven years after disappearance of the virus, clinical signs of HPAI and increased mortality rates were observed among backyard poultry in Kano and in a live bird market in Lagos State, Nigeria. The virus was isolated from 2 samples independently collected from the poultry farm and the market, and H5 subtype virus was identified by reverse transcription PCR. Sequencing of the hemagglutinin (HA) gene showed that the viruses possessed the molecular markers for HPAI viruses with a multibasic amino acid cleavage site motif (PQRERRRKR*G). The complete genome of the virus was submitted to the Global Initiative on Sharing All Influenza Data (GISAID) database and served as reference virus for many cases that were to later follow across the West Africa sub region. The topology of the phylogenetic tree of the HA gene demonstrated that the H5N1 virus from Nigeria (A/chicken/Nigeria/15VIR339-2/2015) falls within genetic clade 2.3.2.1c.

The dynamics of infectious pathogen transmission intra and interspecies have resulted in intercontinental waves of infection in West Africa, and Nigeria especially appears to be a hotspot of HPAI disease outbreaks in the region. In the view of Dr. Meseko, the abundance of different species of animals that inter-mingles in free range, mixed and intensive husbandry with sometimes weak biosecurity is a potential source of emergence of novel pathogens. The opportunity to test this hypothesis was presented with the Award of Alexander von Humboldt postdoctoral research grant hosted by the Freidrich-loeffler-Institut in Germany in 2016. Research done in collaboration with German scientists already showed preliminary results of inter-species transmission of avian influenza to pigs, and has been accepted for publication in *Scientific Reports* (Springer-Nature journals). The study showed the potential for natural exposure and reassortment of avian (H5N1) and human (H1N1pdm09) influenza viruses in pigs (typical mixing vessel).

There have been four pandemics in the last 100 years, the first in 1918 killed about one third of the human population. The fourth pandemic in 2009 was mild yet CDC estimated that between 151,700 and 575,400 people worldwide died in the first year of virus circulation. Both events were caused by viruses that emerged in animals. Scientists are united in their opinion that pandemics are bound to re-occur. Success in control efforts is therefore dependent on how early novel infection is detected before it becomes a catastrophe. A practical approach to achieve this is to monitor emerging pathogens in animals wherein early detection helps to mitigate consequent health and economic impacts.

Dr. Meseko's research objective is to contribute to the ability of the scientific community to detect infection early in its pandemic preparedness through surveillance and monitoring. He also believes that 'the best public health action is before the onset of an epidemic, not during or after'. As part of efforts to share his idea with the global scientific community, he was awarded a travel grant to attend and speak at the 5th International One Health Congress in Saskatoon, Canada in June 2018. Dr. Meseko's scientific life, ideas and work hold many promises for the future in his journey of scientific discovery and quest for solution.

In: Pandemics
Editor: Pavel I. Sidorov

ISBN: 978-1-53614-274-7

Chapter 3

APPLYING PRINCIPLES OF RISK DECISION-MAKING TO INFORM PANDEMIC INFLUENZA PREPAREDNESS AND RESPONSE POLICY

Patrick Saunders-Hastings[1,2,*], PhD,
Lindy Samson[3], MD and Daniel Krewski[1,4], PhD
[1]McLaughlin Centre for Population Health Risk Assessment,
University of Ottawa, Ottawa, ON, Canada
[2]Faculty of Health Sciences, University of Ottawa, Ottawa, ON, Canada
[3]Children's Hospital of Eastern Ontario, Ottawa, ON, Canada
[4]School of Epidemiology, Public Health, and Preventive Medicine,
Faculty of Medicine, University of Ottawa, Ottawa, ON, Canada

ABSTRACT

Influenza pandemics have occurred four times in the past one hundred years, resulting in severe illness, hospitalizations and death

* Corresponding Author Email: patrick.saundershastings@gmail.com.

amongst millions of people. Pandemics can also have serious socioeconomic consequences that disproportionately affect certain population groups. As there is likely to be little time between pandemic virus emergence and global transmission, effective and ethical pandemic preparedness is crucial.

We critically review the most recent Canadian and Ontario pandemic influenza plans, acknowledging that both are currently under revision. Using the principles of public health ethics and risk management, we assess potential avenues for improved pandemic preparedness. In particular, we consider the tensions and trade-offs between different ethical and risk management approaches. Drawing on a taxonomy of regulatory, economic, advisory, community and technological risk management options, we propose intervention strategies at the intersection of ethical and effective risk management practice.

Keywords: pandemic influenza, public health, risk management, risk decision-making, ethics, policy

INTRODUCTION

Influenza infection is caused by an RNA virus which is easily transmitted, leading to annual epidemics of seasonal influenza around the globe (Saunders-Hastings et al. 2016). The clinical spectrum of infection ranges from mild respiratory and systemic symptoms to severe lower respiratory, neurological or systemic illness resulting in hospitalization and death. In otherwise healthy people, typical infection is self-limiting and mild in nature (Lau et al. 2010). However, influenza is currently the most deadly vaccine-preventable disease in North America (Fiore et al. 2008).

Annually, influenza undergoes *antigenic* drift, resulting in a slightly modified virus to which there is residual immunity within the population. Rarely, influenza viruses can undergo an *antigenic shift*, forming a new viral genotype to which humans possess little or no immunity. If this *shifted* virus is efficiently able to transmit between humans and cause significant disease, a global influenza pandemic may occur. This has occurred four times in the past one hundred years. The combined health burden of the 1918 (H1N1) Spanish flu, 1957 (H2N2) Asian flu, 1968

(H3N2) Hong Kong flu and 2009 (H1N1) Swine flu amounts to tens of millions of infections, hospitalizations and deaths (Saunders-Hastings & Krewski 2016). Even the most recent pandemic in 2009 — recognized now as a mild one — is estimated to have resulted in as many as 575,400 global deaths in the first twelve months alone (Dawood et al. 2012). Increasing population density, international travel and viral diversity raise concerns of the possible outbreak of a new influenza pandemic in the near future (Saunders-Hastings & Krewski 2016).

Pandemic influenza can also have serious economic and social consequences. In Canada, worker absenteeism during the 2009 pandemic reached a peak of 9% during the month of November, although this was lower than the peak worker absenteeism of 20–25% expected by Public Health Agency of Canada (Public Health Agency of Canada 2006; Statistics Canada 2010). Total costs associated with the Canadian 2009 pandemic experience have been estimated at approximately CAD $2 billion; direct healthcare costs only accounted for approximately $200 million of this (Canadian Institute for Health Information 2010).

There is a well-documented social gradient of risk with respect to influenza exposure and the experience of adverse outcomes. A literature review of the social determinants of influenza risk reported increased vulnerability among those who were low-income, housing insecure, racial or ethnic minorities, illiterate or of lower educational status, employment insecure or pregnant, as well as those who had limited access to healthcare (O'Sullivan & Bourgoin 2010). In Canada, the need for enhanced targeting of Indigenous groups, migrant workers and immigrants — all of whom tend to be over-represented in terms of influenza hospitalization — has been noted (Garoon & Duggan 2008; Kumar et al. 2009). In developing policy recommendations, it is essential to consider these high-risk groups, in order to avoid an unequal and unfair allocation of resources for protection and treatment.

Age is an important risk factor, with the elderly and the very young tending to be at greater risk from seasonal influenza (Nagata et al. 2013). Pandemic strains, however, typically result in a proportional shift of the health burden towards younger age groups (Saunders-Hastings & Krewski 2016). During the Canadian 2009 H1N1 pandemic, for example, 70% of deaths were in those under 65 years old (Helferty et al. 2010). This can complicate assessment of high-risk age groups for prioritization in intervention design.

The need for effective pandemic preparedness policy has been noted by federal and provincial governments alike, in light of the fact that that there will be little response time between the emergence of a new pandemic strain and its spread into Canada (Ministry of Health and Long-Term Care 2013; Public Health Agency of Canada 2015). Current policies recognize the need for an inter-sectoral, "whole-of-society" approach to pandemic preparedness and response (Public Health Agency of Canada 2015). Identified areas of concern regarding pandemic response capability in Canada include the ability of health systems to accommodate increases in patient demand and maintain adequate supplies of consumables such as vaccines, antivirals and protective equipment (Christian et al. 2006; Cruz et al. 2012; Nap et al. 2007). Failure to meet these challenges could lead to the disruption of essential health and other services, which in turn could have a wide range of negative health, economic and social consequences (Saunders-Hastings et al. 2016).

Given these challenges, it is important that policy planning be based on best practices, as informed by the related fields of public health ethics (PHE) and risk decision-making (RDM). While national and provincial plans assert that they are anchored in these fields, there is little explicit discussion of how the principles of PHE and RDM inform specific intervention strategies, and even less of the tensions and trade-offs that arise from the differential valuation of particular principles. This research aims to fill this knowledge gap.

In subsequent sections, we review existing national and provincial pandemic response plans, examining how PHE and RDM principles might reinforce or alter current practice and leveraging this discussion to inform the proposal of specific intervention strategies. Specifically, we review the national *Canadian Pandemic Influenza Preparedness: Planning Guidance for the Health Sector* and the provincial *Ontario Health Plan for an Influenza Pandemic* (Ministry of Health and Long-Term Care 2013; Public Health Agency of Canada 2015). The Ontario provincial plan was chosen for three reasons: Ontario is the most populated province in Canada; the plan is in its final iteration, and is currently undergoing revision to become the Ontario Influenza Response Plan; and a recent modelling study identified Ontario as the province most vulnerable to influenza-associated surges in patient demand (Saunders-Hastings et al. 2017b).

Table 1. Ten principles of risk decision-making (Jardine et al. 2003; Krewski et al. 2017)

Principle	Definition
1. Risk-based	Allocate resources to optimize return on investment
2. Precautionary principle	In presence of serious threat, act even under situations of substantial uncertainty
3. Balance benefits and risks	In evaluating risk management decisions, evaluate trade-offs in benefits and risks
4. Cost-effectiveness	Seek least cost solution to reduce risk by a given amount
5. Acceptable risk	Accept some level of risk remaining after appropriate management response
6. Zero risk	Seek to entirely eliminate risk
7. Equity	Ensure fair outcomes through an equal distribution of benefits and burdens
8. Stakeholder engagement	Foster opportunities for autonomous participation in decision-making
9. Transparency	Provide full and honest information disclosure to support informed decisions
10. Flexibility	Policies should be flexible to incorporation of new evidence as it becomes available

We draw on the ethical framework of principlism, which promotes principles of justice, autonomy, beneficence and non-malfeasance, to examine collective rights as they relate to utility, equity, proportionality and reciprocity. This is complemented by an analysis of how the ten principles of RDM — elaborated in past publications (Jardine et al. 2003; Krewski et al. 2017) and summarized in Table 1 — provide insight for effective pandemic preparedness and response strategy development. We identify areas of agreement and of tensions in order to propose ways in which future plans may better incorporate these principles to advance ethical and efficient pandemic policy. We propose specific recommendations across the taxonomy of risk management interventions proposed in previous publications, including regulatory, economic, advisory, community and technological measures (Krewski et al. 2007; Krewski et al. 2014).

1. Current Policies

1.1. Canadian Pandemic Influenza Preparedness: Planning Guidance for the Health Sector (CPIP)

CPIP has two primary objectives: to minimize morbidity and mortality and to avoid social disruption resulting from an influenza pandemic (Public Health Agency of Canada 2015). Designed as a guidance document to inform and support response activities of provincial and territorial governments, CPIP recognizes that much of the scope of pandemic response is outside of federal jurisdiction. However, it outlines an inter-sectoral risk management approach to inform provincial and territorial pandemic response. CPIP has been in place since 2004 and is reviewed and updated periodically. This emphasis on RDM was added in the most recent iteration of the plan, with the introduction of impact assessment, pandemic severity scenarios and response triggers (Public Health Agency of Canada 2015).

The plan identifies the need for ethical, equitable and fair decision-making as it relates to the allocation of limited resources such as pandemic vaccine, antiviral medications and hospital resources (Public Health Agency of Canada 2015). Asserting that the determination of equitable allocation will be context-dependent, it clarifies that a focus on collective well-being should take precedence over a narrower clinical focus on individual interests. Other important ethical principles discussed are those of reciprocity and proportionality, discussed in detail in Section 3.1, though there is little discussion of the practical implications of adhering to these principles.

CPIP mentions several important principles of RDM, including transparency, inclusivity and accountability (Public Health Agency of Canada 2015). It supports the iterative "RACE" framework for risk management: recognize, assess, control and evaluate. Other guiding principles discussed include evidence-based decision-making and the precautionary approach; however, there is little discussion of when employing these opposing strategies would be most appropriate. The plan highlights the importance of the effective use of existing surveillance systems, and identifies a gap in the use of mathematical modelling of pandemic flu outbreaks to inform decision-making.

Identified challenges in responding to vulnerable populations include the high provincial disparity in the rural population proportion (Statistics Canada 2015), the high percentage of Indigenous peoples (Statistics Canada 2016) and the high number of recent immigrants in Canada (Statistics Canada 2012). Vulnerable groups are more likely to face challenges in adhering to certain public health recommendations — such as voluntary isolation and hygienic practices — as a result of language and economic barriers (Saunders-Hastings et al. 2017). They may also be less willing and able to access health services. CPIP recognizes that these populations could be marginalized if intervention strategies seek to maximize their reach among the general population, but stops short of proposing targeted strategies for vulnerable and marginalized groups (Public Health Agency of Canada 2015).

A government review of Canadian performance during the 2009 H1N1 pandemic found the response to be satisfactory (Eggleton & Ogilvie 2010). CPIP was credited with effective stockpiling and distribution of vaccines and antivirals and with contributing to a reduction in the overall pandemic burden. Identified weaknesses included a lack of flexibility, scalability and responsiveness to emerging knowledge and pandemic data as it became available (Eggleton & Ogilvie 2010). Recommendations included increased testing of pandemic plans, more effective communication messaging, scaled up data collection and analysis and an increased focus on seasonal influenza preparedness, to be ramped up during a pandemic (Eggleton & Ogilvie 2010). The inclusion of mathematical modelling insights was seen as key to informing the Canadian pandemic response; this constitutes an important bridge which must be further developed moving forward, particularly as it relates to determination of optimal resource allocation (Moghadas et al. 2011). Modelling can inform daily progression of the pandemic, resource-requirement estimates and optimal intervention strategies in situations of uncertainty.

1.2. Ontario Health Plan for an Influenza Pandemic (OHPIP)

Originally released in 2004, OHPIP was in part a reaction to challenges noted in the Toronto response to the 2002 SARS outbreak (Eggleton & Ogilvie 2010; Ministry of Health and Long-Term Care 2013). In its next iteration, OHPIP will be merged into the Ontario Influenza Response Plan (OIRP), an inter-sectoral, disease-specific response document that is currently under development. OIRP will shift the emphasis from pandemic preparedness to the development of a more effective seasonal influenza response, which can be scaled up during a pandemic (Ministry of Health and Long-Term Care 2013). As such, this is an opportune time to assess the strengths and limitations of OHPIP. We do not evaluate in detail the assumption that pandemic challenges will mirror those of seasonal influenza, but do note that flexibility will be crucial to the success of such an approach.

OHPIP shares the objectives outlined by CPIP: minimize illness, death and societal disruption (Ministry of Health and Long-Term Care 2013; Public Health Agency of Canada 2015). With a focus on linking response activities to pandemic severity, OHPIP adheres to the precautionary principle in the absence of reliable epidemiological data (Ministry of Health and Long-Term Care 2013). Though it also identifies evidence-based decision-making as a guiding principle, it does not clarify when or if the latter approach supersedes the former. OHPIP supports health equity, but does not include an ethical framework to support decision-making; the OIRP will include an ethical component, though it is unclear to what extent this will inform the navigation of ethical tensions and resource allocation trade-offs.

OHPIP considers pandemic severity as a product of transmissibility and clinical severity. It embodies the RDM principle of transparent stakeholder engagement. In the new OIRP, the Ontario Ministry of Health and Long-term Care (MOHLTC) will seek to improve communication strategies, especially as they relate to vulnerable populations, social media and health systems (Ministry of Health and Long-Term Care 2013). Identified gap areas include a lack of substantive discussion regarding the role of predictive modelling to improve risk-based preparedness efforts through surveillance, cost-effectiveness assessment and identification of vulnerable health systems (Ministry of Health and Long-Term Care 2013).

The province of Ontario must accommodate vulnerable groups similar to those identified in CPIP; these include rural populations, Indigenous peoples and immigrants. OHPIP also recognises those with substance addiction, the homeless and those without a primary care provider as vulnerable populations (Ministry of Health and Long-Term Care 2013). The focus throughout this guidance is on accessing hard-to-reach populations and protecting essential service delivery in emergency situations.

In Ontario, public health functions are performed by municipal or county boards appointed by municipalities and provinces (Eggleton & Ogilvie 2010). In the aftermath of the 2009 H1N1 pandemic, representatives were asked to evaluate Ontario's response. Criticisms included inadequate distribution of vaccine supplies to meet demand and barriers to inter-sectoral and inter-jurisdictional collaboration (Eggleton & Ogilvie 2010). A key point of focus was the need for a more flexible, proportionate response that could be scaled up and down as the pandemic evolved; this would support principle-based planning that avoids overreliance on planning assumptions that may prove to be inaccurate.

2. Principle-Based Approaches

2.1. Public Health Ethics

CPIP proposes that, in a pandemic emergency, collective rights should take priority over individual ones, promoting the principles of utility (maximizing benefit), proportionality (measured response), reciprocity (assisting individuals and community in discharge of duties) and equity and distributive justice (fair distribution of resources, benefits and burdens) (Public Health Agency of Canada 2015). OHPIP adopts similar principles, supplementing them with principles of individual liberty, privacy and duty to provide care (University of Toronto Joint Centre for Bioethics Pandemic Influenza Working Group 2005). Both plans support the building of trust and solidarity (Ministry of Health and Long-Term Care 2013; Public Health Agency of Canada 2009). However, these principles do not in themselves constitute a framework, and provide little procedural or strategic insight.

In this section we examine pandemic policy within the classic ethical framework of principlism, based on four keys to ethical public health practice: justice, beneficence, non-malfeasance and autonomy (Callahan 2003). It has been argued that autonomy and justice should be the central focus, as any infringement on them would compromise the principles of beneficence and non-malfeasance (Callahan 2003). If we consider beneficence to include the collective good of the community, and non-malfeasance the avoidance of infringement on social and political values, it becomes evident that violating justice or autonomy would compromise both of these ideals. Following this argument, we will suggest that prioritizing justice and autonomy should guide our assessments of ethical pandemic policy. We therefore focus on these two principles, and discuss beneficence and non-malfeasance within the contexts of justice, autonomy and — in the subsequent section — risk management.

The strength of such a principle-based ethical framework is its simplicity and readiness for application to practice. However, the suitability of principlism for the assessment of ethics in public health has been called into question, as it is more traditionally viewed in the context of individualistic clinical ethics (Callahan 2003). Upshur, for example, sought to shift the discussion of public health ethics to four more collective principles: the harm principle, least restrictive means principle, reciprocity principle and transparency principle (Upshur 2002). The harm principle, as set out by John Stuart Mill, asserts that the only ethical infringement upon individual liberty is to prevent harm to others (Mill 1959). The least restrictive means principle proposes that more coercive methods should only be initiated once less severe interventions have failed (Coker 2001). The reciprocity principle assigns responsibility to social organizations to assist individuals and communities in performing their ethical duties (Harris & Holm 1995). The transparency principle holds that all stakeholders should be involved in an open decision-making process.

We do not view this discussion as indicative that principlism is inappropriate, but rather as an extension of its principles to the collective ideals of justice and autonomy, allowing their application to community settings. We therefore conclude this section with a review of these two pillars of principlism and how they relate to those presented by Upshur and by CPIP.

2.1.1. Justice

Justice requires an assessment of what constitutes an appropriate distribution of limited resources. In conventional medical ethics, "need" is often viewed as the most important factor, where there is a moral imperative to treat as many people as possible (Metz 2008). This becomes more complicated in emergency situations, where resources are limited and may have to be distributed preferentially. For example, modelling studies have suggested that pandemic-associated increases in patient demand could require 7.5–19.5% of acute-care bed capacity in Canada and over 100% of ICU capacity, even under moderate disease assumptions (Christian et al. 2006; Saunders-Hastings et al. 2017a; Saunders-Hastings et al. 2017b). Given already high bed occupancy rates, this would likely necessitate a diversion of hospital resources, causing service disruption. The "priority" argument would support acting in a utilitarian way so as to maximize the number of lives saved, even if such an approach would mean a disruption of services for other groups or diseases (Metz 2008). This is reflected in the primary CPIP and OHPIP objectives, and supports triage of patients to prioritize those most likely to recover within the shortest amount of time. It could also be invoked to support preferential investment in urban settings, which are likely to experience more transmission than rural areas.

Criticisms of the priority argument could be based upon two other ethical arguments. The Kantian "equality argument" states that all lives should be considered of equal value, and prioritizing certain individuals is unjust (Metz 2008). The Rawlsian theory of justice proposes that priority should be given to those that are worst off (Rawls 1971). Both arguments are consistent with an approach that prioritizes saving lives, but they shift the discussion towards the prioritization of life-saving treatments over prevention, despite the fact that prevention may save more lives overall. They also suggest that those at increased risk of adverse health outcomes may have a stronger claim to resources than those more likely to experience uncomplicated infection, but that preference should not be given based upon income level or location alone. This has implications for the prioritization of therapeutic treatment over prophylaxis, and limiting access to critical care to those who require mechanical ventilation. Such trade-offs highlight the tensions that may arise between utility and equity in emergency situations. These principles also refocus the discussion of resource allocation and triage decisions upon the implications of treatment for chances of survival and future quality of life, and recognizes as unjust the consideration of other intrinsic characteristics such as age, gender, race, religion, socioeconomic status, geographic location or existence of a disability (Ministry of Health and Long-Term Care 2008).

Another important issue regarding the distribution of limited resources involves whether preferential access to protective measures should be granted to healthcare workers; this relates closely to the reciprocity principle, introduced above. CPIP supports the reciprocity principle, wherein social organizations like public health systems are morally responsible to support those who might incur risks as a result of the discharge of their responsibilities. In the context of pandemic influenza, this is most commonly associated with giving the highest priority to healthcare workers, who may be at increased risk of infection. The "responsibility argument" might advocate against this, suggesting that such an approach fails to hold people accountable for their actions, as proper adherence to personal protective protocols should adequately protect healthcare workers from risks in excess of those in the general population (Metz 2008). Utilitarian views, however, are likely to support the reciprocity principle in this case, as protection of healthcare workers has the indirect benefit of limiting transmission among their patients — who may be at increased risk of complications — and minimizing the risk of health service disruption as a result of worker absenteeism. It should also be noted that healthcare providers are at risk of infection in home and community settings, where they are unlikely to be in protective equipment, and therefore their protection becomes an important component of promoting service continuity.

2.1.2. Autonomy

Autonomy involves giving individuals maximum liberty to make decisions that will affect their health. In conventional medical ethics the focus tends to be on a patient or study subject, supporting procedures such as informed consent. The public health transparency principle, advocating for open stakeholder engagement, is a logical extension of autonomy (Upshur 2002). The harm and least restrictive means principles similarly support autonomy, recognizing a duty to minimize infringement upon individual liberty. In the context of current pandemic plans, the principle of proportionality supports tailoring the intensity of intervention strategies to the severity of the pandemic scenario, avoiding mandatory or costly interventions as much as possible.

These principles are relevant to communication strategies and mandatory public health measures — such as school closure, workplace closure or quarantine — initiated during influenza pandemics. Open communication is crucial to fostering public trust, uptake of public health recommendations and appropriate resource use (O'Malley et al. 2009). Strategies must also avoid exclusively addressing the disease, to the exclusion of population considerations. Such a paternalistic approach can undermine communication efforts, obstructing achievement of optimal health outcomes, especially among populations that are already marginalized (Verweij 2009). Some areas, such as Toronto, Ontario, are developing all-hazards communication and response strategies specific to particular vulnerable groups; such an effort would support the transparency principle in a way that is also likely to advance justice, beneficence and non-malfeasance (City of Toronto 2015; 2017).

The harm and least restrictive means principles may be of particular relevance to regulations surrounding antiviral prophylaxis. Increasing access to antiviral prophylaxis could deplete stockpiled drug availability for treatment, thereby limiting access to treatment options among infected individuals in the future. The potential benefit of containing an early-stage pandemic must also be weighed against the ethical obligation to ensure that drug resistance does not emerge. Contact tracing and distribution of prophylactics may also occur disproportionately in easy-to-access population groups, such as healthcare workers, which may lead to a further service access imbalance among vulnerable groups. In this scenario, the harm principle and least restrictive means principle seem to support opposing strategies, wherein the harm principle supports restriction of individual access to prophylaxis; in contrast, the least restrictive means principle might oppose such infringement upon individual liberty unless absolutely necessary. However, the moral imperative to protect and save as many lives as possible, even if this results in some limitation of individual liberties, suggests that individuals should not be allowed to develop personal stockpiles of protective consumables.

2.2. Risk Decision-Making Principles

Of the ten principles of RDM, four relate closely to ethical principles discussed in the previous section. Equity, stakeholder engagement, transparency and flexibility reflect the ethical principles of justice, autonomy and proportionality that are important to almost any public health intervention. As such, these are only discussed briefly, given the more thorough analysis in the previous section. We focus our discussion on the tensions between three pairs of related RDM principles as they relate to pandemic policy: risk-based decision-making and the precautionary principle; risk-benefit and cost-effectiveness; and acceptable risk and zero risk tolerance.

2.2.1. Risk-Based Decision-Making and the Precautionary Principle

Risk-based decision-making supports the allocation of resources to maximize risk reduction for a given investment, while the precautionary principle supports action to mitigate a serious threat, even under situations of uncertainty (Jardine et al. 2003). As influenza pandemics are potentially catastrophic events that are inherently uncertain — where the disease characteristics cannot be known in advance of emergence — plans tend to support a precautionary approach, particularly in the early stages of an outbreak (Ministry of Health and Long-Term Care 2013; Public Health Agency of Canada 2015). This raises questions, however, about the point at which emerging data are sufficient to support a transition to risk-based decision-making, and presents challenges in scaling community and health system responses to pandemic severity. Indeed, a key challenge identified during the 2009 H1N1 pandemic was in adjusting response efforts to pandemic severity as the pandemic developed and dissipated (Eggleton & Ogilvie 2010).

While high uncertainty and potential consequences justify the precautionary principle in the planning and early stages of a pandemic, it is crucial to invoke risk-based decision-making as early as possible. This could involve the expanded adoption of inter-pandemic mathematical modelling, as well as scaling up surveillance efforts to capitalize on emerging technologies. Planners must acknowledge that pandemic assumptions are likely to be inaccurate, and that an over-reliance on inaccurate assumptions could result in disproportionate response efforts. A principle-based planning and response mandate would facilitate flexibility and the incorporation of empirical data as it became available.

2.2.2. Risk-Benefit and Cost-Effectiveness

Both the risk-benefit and cost-effectiveness principles seek to evaluate interventions across a standardized calculation of benefits and costs. The risk-benefit principle advocates for the evaluation of trade-offs in intervention strategies, suggesting that efforts should be made to maximize benefits and minimize hazards. The cost-effectiveness principle advocates for pursuing the least-cost intervention to reduce risk by a given amount (Weinstein & Stason 1977). These principles are often prioritized in pandemic influenza preparedness planning, where resources are likely to become scarce and many lives are at stake; this is evident in the utilitarian primary objective to save as many lives as possible (Public Health Agency of Canada 2015).

However, an over-reliance on such an economical approach can be problematic in a number of ways. First, if we accept that health outcomes can be aggregated and calculated in economic terms, we face challenges in assigning values to given outcomes, particularly mortality. Some government valuations of life have ranged between six and nine million dollars (USD) (Appelbaum 2011). Other analyses assign a value for each life-year lost (LYL); in Canada, CAD$ 50,000 per life-year saved is the commonly accepted threshold for an effective intervention (Winquist et al. 2012). Second, once we accept that life can be measured in economic terms, there is a space to argue that the dire needs of a few can be outweighed by the smaller needs of many, or by the economic cost of intervening (Verweij 2009). This can lead to a prioritization of mass prevention, particularly among younger age groups in urban locations, where there is the potential to increase life-years saved. While this is an important component of pandemic response, it would be unethical to scale prevention to an extent that it disrupts treatment-side service delivery, or prevention services in hard-to-reach populations. Lastly, the argument can be made that non-health risks and benefits should be excluded from risk-benefit analysis, and instead only included in cost-effectiveness analyses of intervention strategies with similar risk-benefit ratios and equity impacts (Verweij 2009).

2.2.3. Acceptable Risk and Zero Risk

The principle of acceptable risk acknowledges that the complete elimination of risk may not be feasible, and that some will remain even after the appropriate implementation of intervention strategies; the zero risk principle supports efforts to eradicate risk entirely (Hunter & Fewtrell 2001; Krewski et al. 2008). In the context of pandemic influenza, few would suggest that zero risk is an attainable goal, as some level of residual risk seems unavoidable. This is rarely explicitly stated, however, and levels of acceptable risk in pandemic situations are unclear.

Public and organizational risk acceptability will have important implications for early containment efforts and the thresholds for triggering emergency measures such as school and work closure and quarantine protocols. It is also of relevance to worker absenteeism, which can exacerbate pandemic-related economic burden and essential service disruption (House et al. 2011; Mitchell et al. 2012; Nap et al. 2007). Open communication strategies can foster public trust, facilitate effective emergency protocols, and reduce worker absenteeism. Risk management strategies should not pursue a "zero risk" strategy. Rather, an important component of preparedness should be communication efforts to support knowledge and acceptance of some form of unavoidable risk level.

2.2.4. Equity, Stakeholder Engagement, Transparency and Flexibility

Equity in risk management refers to the promotion of a fair and proportionate distribution of risks, benefits and costs. Stakeholder engagement and transparency acknowledge the importance of the active involvement of — and open communication with — interested parties. These are essential to policy decisions in democratic societies, and can improve risk reduction outcomes by promoting community trust and adherence with risk management recommendations. Flexibility centres upon the ability to incorporate new risk information to inform decision-making. These four principles can be viewed as the ethical foundation of RDM, and are important considerations for almost all risk reduction efforts. These principles relate closely to the ethical principles of justice, autonomy and proportionality discussed in the previous section. We will therefore refrain from restating their policy implications and trade-offs with other principles, and instead emphasize the congruence between principles of PHE and RDM. Principles from both domains are incorporated into our strategic recommendations below.

3. Strategic Recommendations

The previous sections have set out examples of pandemic plans in Canada, presenting principles of PHE and RDM that should inform strategic and procedural development and updating of these plans. Below, we review how these principles could direct ethical and effective strategies across a range of public health interventions.

3.1. Regulatory Interventions

Principles of autonomy, proportionality and least restrictive means would support efforts to minimize regulatory interventions, employing them only where absolutely necessary. Whereas government or international health regulations, such as surveillance reporting and adherence to best practices, are important components of pandemic preparedness, regulations on individual citizens should be avoided where possible. Currently, in low-transmissibility or low-severity pandemic scenarios, the only mandatory measure proposed by OHPIP is contact tracing and case management; only in a pandemic that is both highly transmissible and clinically severe is it suggested that other mandatory measures may be required (Ministry of Health and Long-Term Care 2013).

Taken together, this would suggest that interventions such as mandatory quarantine and school closure should be avoided unless the pandemic is extremely severe and they are accompanied by other control measures. There is little public support for these interventions, and a systematic review of pandemics to date found little evidence of significant impact or cost-effectiveness (Baum et al. 2009; Blendon et al. 2006; Garrett et al. 2009; Saunders-Hastings et al., 2016). Similarly, a modelling study found that voluntary isolation of infected individuals is more cost-effective, and does not infringe upon individual liberty (Saunders-Hastings et al. 2017a). Most interventions should be focused across the other four categories. However, there are two key issues where regulation could promote pandemic preparedness.

First, while some might suggest that antivirals be made available without prescriptions during influenza pandemics, in order to reduce patient inflow and transmission in healthcare settings, this should be avoided as it could lead to personal stockpiling, over-reliance on general antiviral prophylaxis and an accumulation of drug-resistant viral strains. Instead, prescriptions should be available via pharmacists and telemedicine, which supports risk reduction and principles of justice and non-malfeasance. Where antiviral prophylaxis is implemented, thresholds should be established *a priori* to determine the groups that will be subject to contact tracing and prophylaxis, and at what point this is to be cut off, with an emphasis on preserving stockpiles for case treatment throughout multiple waves.

Second, regulations based upon the reciprocity principle must be considered based upon quantifiable risk. While ethical principles support the provision of protection to healthcare workers that may be at increased risk, there is a need to base this on empirical data. In the past, those in direct contact with patients — such as healthcare providers and room-cleaning staff — have been prioritized. However, little is known about how the risk levels of these groups differ from those of other healthcare-associated staff (such as administrative staff) or the general public, which may not have equivalent access to protective equipment (Verweij 2009). Measures to protect healthcare workers are needed, but should be grounded in risk, cost-effectiveness and equity assessments. Meanwhile, increasing knowledge of existing emergency plans has been identified as a gap in current plans, with one study finding a need for more training and information for Canadian healthcare workers (O'Sullivan et al. 2008).

3.2. Economic Interventions

Economic interventions are a critical component of any plan, as resources are likely to be limited in pandemic situations and the potential economic burden is high. Cost-effective interventions such as vaccination, antiviral use, personal protective measures and voluntary isolation should be promoted over school closure, community-contact reduction and quarantine, which can dramatically increase economic burden with relatively little impact on transmission or overall pandemic burden (Saunders-Hastings et al. 2016; Saunders-Hastings et al. 2017a).

Economic interventions should seek to reduce the economic barriers to intervention uptake. This is important to support principles of equity, distributive justice and beneficence, for lack of resource access can influence disease exposure, capacity to protect oneself from exposure and capacity to adhere to guidelines during infection. Lower income individuals, for example, may not be able to comply with voluntary isolation guidelines that suggest staying home from work, which could lead to lost income and job insecurity (Baum et al. 2009; Blumenshine et al. 2008).

The same is true for individuals that may be required to stay home to care for a sick family member or a child sent home due to school closure

(Bouye et al. 2009; O'Sullivan et al. 2009). While business continuity plans are not explicitly addressed in CPIP or OHPIP, further consideration of economic interventions to support flexible work patterns is needed; these may include encouraging employers to support policies such as telecommuting or special pay subsidies for those required to miss work.

Similar findings of low vaccine coverage among low-income groups suggest a possible benefit of economic incentives among high-risk groups. One study found that social assistance and seniors' benefits increased vaccination rates among low-income groups during the Canadian 2009 H1N1 experience (Hobbs & Buxton 2014). Vaccination and voluntary isolation are among the most effective and cost-effective interventions available, with high benefit-risk ratios; economic interventions have an important role in supporting equitable expansion of their adherence (Saunders-Hastings et al. 2016).

3.3. Advisory Interventions

Advisory interventions provide accurate and timely information about health risks and how to avoid them, as well as justifications for policy decisions (Krewski et al. 2007). Thus, advisory interventions will centre upon effective, transparent and equitable communication messaging strategies. A crucial component of these efforts will be the engagement of vulnerable groups. Efforts should be made to ensure that all groups — especially those that are high-risk or hard-to reach — receive information on pandemic risks and available interventions (Truman et al. 2009). This could involve working with vulnerable groups to collect specialized data, explicitly addressing population concerns (such as vaccine hesitancy) in public health messaging and the development of multi-media campaign platforms that are accessible to people of different languages, cultures and literacy levels (Truman et al. 2009). While general public health messaging is important and may reach more individuals, targeting of vulnerable groups is crucial to supporting trust, autonomy and uptake among populations that may be at increased risk of developing complicated infections, thereby supporting equitable and effective risk reduction.

3.4. Community Interventions

Community interventions involve the empowerment of citizens to participate in priority-setting, decision-making, planning and implementation (Krewski et al. 2007). Successful and ethical advisory interventions require bidirectional communication, and active stakeholder engagement is crucial to supporting uptake and autonomy among vulnerable groups. Engaging community leaders and organizations — as well as members of vulnerable and marginalized populations — builds trust and credibility among communities that are sometimes suspicious of healthcare professionals (Poland 2010). Key components of planning in this area could include the involvement of faith- and community-based organizations in plans to disseminate information, both to public health organizations and to their service population (Truman et al. 2009). Such organizations could advise planners on effective communication strategies, act as education and service provision centers, and assist in surveillance efforts. Such efforts would support autonomy, uptake, local ownership and cost-effective health protection campaigns.

3.5. Technological Interventions

Technological interventions rely on innovation to improve response capacity and flexibility (Krewski et al. 2007). With respect to pandemic influenza, this may be most relevant to considerations of what kinds of evidence are incorporated into surveillance and decision-making processes. First, the popularity of social media holds promise for an expansion of real-time surveillance efforts. Second, mathematical modelling, in conjunction with a principle-based approach, can be useful in providing a proxy for risk-based decision-making in the absence of reliable epidemiological data. The continuous development of complex and technologically advanced models can facilitate flexibility and responsiveness of intervention strategies as new data emerge. Lastly, advances in hospital electronic records and regional partnership could help inter-hospital collaboration to maximize resource use efficiency and promote regional hospital-resource adequacy. Another important consideration is the development, acceleration and then maintenance of vaccine manufacturing technology. This has important implications for the speed of deployment and population coverage achieved in the early stages of a pandemic, and should be encouraged alongside efforts to promote more equitable international vaccine distribution. It should be noted that new technologies may not always be supportive of ethical and risk management principles, raising new questions and trade-offs. It will be important to ensure that technological strategies adhere to public health and risk management principles, and that there is a space for continued discussion of what and how principles should be prioritized in new contexts.

CONCLUSION

In the present paper, we consider Canadian pandemic preparedness through the lenses of public health ethics and risk management. While national and provincial plans make reference to a range of principles, there is limited discussion of how these might inform strategic and procedural directions. As plans are currently being revised and updated, this work presents a timely discussion of the tensions between different strategic policy options.

Specifically, we review the *Canadian Pandemic Influenza Plan* and *Ontario Health Plan for an Influenza Pandemic*. We note trade-offs between different principles, but emphasize that there is substantial compatibility between the two domains, and a space for policy interventions positioned at the intersection of ethical and effective risk management practice.

We propose a range of intervention principles and strategies to improve pandemic preparedness. Specific recommendations promote caution in implementing mandatory public health measures, risk-based prioritization of healthcare workers and the uptake of — and capacity to adhere to — pubic health recommendations, particularly among vulnerable groups. Lastly, planners should use caution in rolling out antiviral prophylaxis, and pandemic severity thresholds for discontinuation should be established *a priori*.

Future research should seek to combine empirical data with mathematical modelling to inform risk-based policy decisions, particularly as they relate to thresholds for action, population group prioritization and resource-planning. There is also a space for deeper consideration of the ethical implications of emerging technology as it applies to pandemic preparedness.

REFERENCES

Appelbaum, B. (2011). As U.S. agencies put more value on a life, businesses fret. *The New York Times*. Retrieved from http://www.nytimes.com/2011/02/17/business/economy/17regulation.html?_r=0.

Baum, N., Jacobson, P. & Goold, D. (2009). "Listen to the people": public deliberation about social distancing measures in a pandemic. *American Journal of Bioethics*. 9(11): 4-14.

Blendon, R., DesRoches, C., Cetron, M., Benson, J., Meinhardt, T. & Pollard, W. (2006). Attitudes toward the use of quarantine in a public health emergency in four countries. *Health affairs*. 25(2): w15-25.

Blumenshine, P., Reingold, A., Egerter, S., Mockenhaupt, R., Braveman, P., & Marks, J. (2008). Pandemic influenza planning in the United States from a health disparities perspective. *Emerging infectious diseases*. 14(5): 709-715.

Bouye, K., Truman, B., Hutchins, S., Richard, R., Brown, C., Guillory, J. & Rashid, J. (2009). Pandemic Influenza preparedness and response among public-housing residents, single-parent families, and low-income populations. *American journal of public health.* 99(S2): S287-293.

Callahan, D. (2003). Principlism and communitarianism. *Journal of medical ethics.* 29(5): 287-291.

Christian, M., Hawryluck, L., Wax, R., Cook, T., Lazar, N., Herridge, M., Burkle, F. (2006). Development of a triage protocol for critical care during an influenza pandemic. *CMAJ.* 175(11): 1377-1381.

Canadian Institute for Health Information. (2010). The Impact of the H1N1 Pandemic on Canadian hospitals. Retrieved from https://secure.cihi.ca/estore/productSeries.htm?pc=PCC545.

City of Toronto. (2015). *The Toronto Seniors Strategy*: Towards an Age-Friendly City. Retrieved from https://www1.toronto.ca/City%20Of%20Toronto/Social%20Development,%20Finance%20&%20Administration/Shared%20Content/Seniors/PDFs/seniors-strategy-fullreport.pdf.

City of Toronto. (2017). *Toronto Newcomer Strategy.* Retrieved from http://www.toronto.ca/legdocs/mmis/2013/cd/bgrd/backgroundfile-55333.pdf.

Coker, R. (2001). Detentions and mandatory treatment for tuberculosis in Russia. *Lancet.* 358(9279): 349-350.

Cruz, A., Tittle, K., Smith, E. & Sirbaugh, P. (2012). Increasing out-of-hospital regional surge capacity for H1N1 2009 influenza a through existing community pediatrician offices: a qualitative description of quality improvement strategies. *Disaster medicine and public health preparedness.* 6(2): 113-116.

Dawood, F., Luliano, D., Reed, C., Meltzer, M., Shay, D., Cheng, P., Widdowson, M. (2012). Estimated global mortality associated with the first 12 months of 2009 pandemic influenza A H1N1 virus circulation: a modelling study. *Lancet infectious diseases.* 12(9): 687-695.

Eggleton, A. & Ogilvie, K. (2010). *Canada's response to the 2009 H1N1 influenza pandemic.* Ottawa, ON: Senate of Canada.

Fiore, A., Shay, D., Broder, K., Iskander, J., Uyeki, T., Mootrey, G., Cox, N. (2008). Prevention and control of influenza: recommendations of the Advisory Committee on Immunization Practices (ACIP), 2008. *Morbidity and mortality weekly report.* 57: 1-60.

Garoon, J. & Duggan, P. (2008). Discourses of disease, discourses of disadvantage: a critical analysis of National Pandemic Influenza Preparedness Plans. *Social science & medicine*. 67(7): 1133-1142.

Garrett, J., Vawter, D., Prehn, A., DeBruin, D. & Gervais, K. (2009). Listen! The value of public engagement in pandemic ethics. *American journal of bioethics*. 9(11): 17-19.

Harris, J. & Holm, S. (1995). Is there a moral obligation not to infect others? *BMJ*. 311(7014): 1215-1217.

Helferty, M., Vachon, J., Tarasuk, J., Rodin, R., Spika, J. & Pelletier, L. (2010). Incidence of hospital admissions and severe outcomes during the first and second waves of pandemic (H1N1) 2009. *CMAJ*. 182(18): 1981-1987.

Hobbs, J. & Buxton, J. (2014). Influenza immunization in Canada's low-income population. *BMC public health*. 14(1): 740.

House, T., Baguelin, M., Van Hoek, A., White, P., Sadique, Z., Eames, K., Keeling, M. (2011). Modelling the impact of local reactive school closures on critical care provision during an influenza pandemic. *Proceedings of the royal society B: biological sciences*. 278(1719): 2753-2760.

Hunter, P. R., & Fewtrell, L. (2001). Acceptable risk. *Water Quality: Guidelines, Standards and Health Risk assessment and management for water-related infectious disease*. London, UK: World Health Organisation.

Jardine, C., Hrudey, S., Shortreed, J., Craig, L., Krewski, D., Furgal, C. & McColl, S. (2003). Risk management frameworks for human health and environmental risks. *Journal of toxicology and environmental health part B*. 6(6): 569-720.

Krewski, D., Hogan, V., Turner, M., Zeman, P., McDowell, I., Edwards, N. & Losos, J. (2007). An Integrated Framework for Risk Management and Population Health. *Human and ecological risk assessment: an international journal.* 13(6): 1288-1312.

Krewski, D., Lemyre, L., Turner, M., Lee, J., Dallaire, C., Bouchard, L., Mercier, P. (2008). Public perception of population health risks in

Canada: Risk perception beliefs. *Health, risk & society*. 10(2): 167-179.

Krewski, D., Saunders-Hastings, P., Westphal, M., Leiss, W., Dusseault, M., Gray, G., Attaran, A. (2017). Ten principles of risk decision-making. *Environmental health perspectives*. In preparation.

Krewski, D., Westphal, M., Andersen, M., Paoli, G., Chiu, W., Al-Zoughool, M., Cote, I. (2014). A framework for the next generation of risk science. *Environmental health perspectives*. 122(8): 796-805.

Kumar, A., Zarychanski, R., Pinto, R., Cook, D., Marshall, J., Lacroix, J. & Stelfox, T. (2009). Critically ill patients with 2009 influenza A (H1N1) infection in Canada. *JAMA*. 302(17): 1872-1879.

Lau, J., Griffiths, S., Choi, K. & Lin, C. (2010). Prevalence of preventive behaviors and associated factors during early phase of the H1N1 influenza epidemic. *American journal of infection control*. 38(5): 374-380.

Metz, T. (2008). Respect for persons permits prioritizing treatment for HIV/AIDS. *Developing world bioethics*. 8(2): 89-103.

Mill, J. (1959). *On liberty*. Landam, MD, USA: University Press America.

Mitchell, R., Ogunremi, T., Astrakianakis, G., Bryce, E., Gervais, R., Gravel, D., Weir, C. (2012). Impact of the 2009 influenza A (H1N1) pandemic on Canadian health care workers: A survey on vaccination, illness, absenteeism, and personal protective equipment. *American journal of infection control*. 40(7): 611-616.

Moghadas, S., Pizzi, N., Wu, J., Tamblyn, S., & Fisman, D. (2011). Canada in the face of the 2009 H1N1 pandemic. *Influenza and other respiratory viruses*. 5(2): 83-88.

Ministry of Health and Long-Term Care. (2008). *The Ontario Health Plan for an Influenza Pandemic*. Toronto, ON: MOHLTC.

Ministry of Health and Long-Term Care. (2013). *Ontario Health Plan for an Influenza Pandemic*. Toronto, Canada: MOHLTC.

Nagata, J., Hernández-Ramos, I., Kurup, A., Albrecht, D., Vivas-Torrealba, C. & Franco-Paredes, C. (2013). Social determinants of health and seasonal influenza vaccination in adults ≥65 years: a systematic review of qualitative and quantitative data. *BMC public health.* 13(1): 388.

Nap, R., Andriessen, P., Meesen, N. & Werf, T. (2007). Pandemic influenza and hospital resources. *Emerging infectious diseases.* 13(11): 1714-1719.

O'Malley, P., Rainford, J. & Thompson, A. (2009). Transparency during public health emergencies: from rhetoric to reality. *Bulletin of the World Health Organization.* 87: 614-618.

O'Sullivan, T., Amaratunga, C., Phillips, K., Coneil, W., O'Connor, E., Lemyre, L. & Dow, D. (2009). If Schools Are Closed, Who Will Watch Our Kids? Family Caregiving and Other Sources of Role Conflict among Nurses During Large Scale Outbreaks. *Prehospital disaster medicine.* 24(4): 321-325.

O'Sullivan, T. & Bourgoin, M. (2010). *Vulnerability in an influenza pandemic: Looking beyond the medical risk.* Ottawa, Canada: International Centre for Infectious Diseases.

O'Sullivan, T., Dow, D., Turner, M., Lemyre, L., Corneil, W., Krewski, D., Amaratunga, C. (2008). Disaster and emergency management: Canadian nurses' perceptions of preparedness on hospital front lines. *Prehospital disaster medicine.* 23(3): s11-18.

Public Health Agency of Canada (2006). *Canadian Pandemic Influenza Plan for the Health Sector.* Ottawa, Canada: PHAC.

Public Health Agency of Canada. (2009). *Canadian Pandemic Influenza Preparedness: Planning Guidance for the Health Sector.* Ottawa, Canada: PHAC.

Public Health Agency of Canada (2015). *Canadian Pandemic Influenza Preparedness: Planning Guidance for the Health Sector.* Ottawa, Canada: PHAC.

Poland, G. (2010). The 2009-2010 influenza pandemic: effects on pandemic and seasonal vaccine uptake and lessons learned for seasonal vaccination campaigns. *Vaccine.* 28(s4): 3–13.

Rawls, J. (1971). *Theory of justice.* Oxford, UK: Oxford University Press.

Saunders-Hastings, P., Crispo, J., Sikora, L. & Krewski, D. (2017). Effectiveness of personal protective measures in reducing pandemic influenza transmission: a systematic review and meta-analysis. *Epidemics*. 20:1–20.

Saunders-Hastings, P. & Krewski, D. (2016). Reviewing the History of Pandemic Influenza: Understanding Patterns of Emergence and Transmission. *Pathogens*. 5(66).

Saunders-Hastings, P., Quinn Hayes, B., Smith, R. & Krewski, D. (2017a). Modelling community-control strategies to protect hospital resources during a pandemic influenza in Ottawa, Canada. *PLOS one*. 12(6): e0179315.

Saunders-Hastings, P., Quinn Hayes, B., Smith, R. & Krewski, D. (2017b). National assessment of Canadian pandemic preparedness: employing InFluNet to identify high-risk areas for inter-wave vaccine distribution. *Infectious Disease Modelling*. 2(3):341–352.

Saunders-Hastings, P., Reisman, J. & Krewski, D. (2016). Assessing the State of Knowledge Regarding the Effectiveness of Interventions to Contain Pandemic Influenza Transmission: A Systematic Review and Narrative Synthesis. *PLOS one*. 11(12): e0168262.

Statistics Canada. (2010). *Impact of H1N1 and seasonal flu on hours worked.* Retrieved from http://www.statcan.gc.ca/daily-quotidien/100115/dq100115c-eng.htm.

Statistics Canada. (2012). *Canada Year Book*, 2012. Retrieved from http://www.statcan.gc.ca/pub/11-402-x/11-402-x2012000-eng.htm.

Statistics Canada. (2015). *Canada's rural population since 1851.* Retrieved from https://www12.statcan.gc.ca/census-recensement/2011/as-sa/98-310-x/98-310-x2011003_2-eng.cfm.

Statistics Canada. (2016). *Aboriginal Peoples in Canada: First Nations People, Métis and Inuit.* Retrieved from https://www12.statcan.gc.ca/nhs-enm/2011/as-sa/99-011-x/99-011-x2011001-eng.cfm.

Truman, B., Tinker, T., Vaughan, E., Kapella, B., Brenden, M., Woznica, C., Lichtveld, M. (2009). Pandemic Influenza Preparedness and Response among Immigrants and Refugees. *American journal of public health*. 99(Suppl 2): S278-S286.

University of Toronto Joint Centre for Bioethics Pandemic Influenza Working Group. (2005). "Stand on Guard for thee." *Ethical considerations in preparedness planning for pandemic influenza.* Toronto, Canada: University of Toronto.

Upshur, R. (2002). Principles for the justification of public health intervention. *Canadian journal of public health.* 93(2): 101-103.

Verweij, M. (2009). Moral Principles for Allocating Scarce Medical Resources in an Influenza Pandemic. *Journal of bioethical inquiry.* 6(2):159-169.

Weinstein, M. & Stason, W. (1977). Foundations of cost-effectiveness analysis for health and medical practices. *New England journal of medicine.* 296: 716-721.

Winquist, E., Bell, C., Clarke, J., Evans, G., Martin, J., Sabharwal, M., Coyle, D. (2012). An evaluation framework for funding drugs for rare diseases. *Value in health.* 15(6): 982-986.

Biographical Sketch

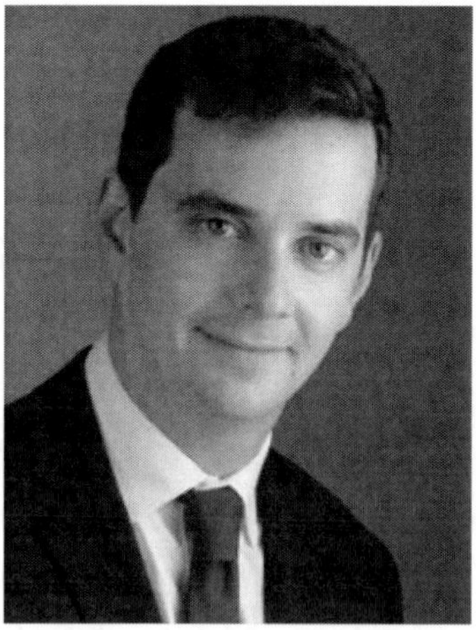

Dr. Patrick Saunders-Hastings is an epidemiologist and health informatics consultant working in the Gevity Population and Public Health Practice. With expertise in health information systems, infectious disease epidemiology and environmental health, Patrick combines qualitative and quantitative methodologies to inform strategies, programs and decisions designed to improve health outcomes.

Patrick's research interests include infectious disease preparedness, climate change adaptation and the use of information and communication technologies to improve health. He supports evidence-based decision-making for clients from the public and private sector. A few of his past projects have included safety and effectiveness assessments of pharmaceutical products, national implementations of health information systems and technical services to support climate change adaptation projects.

Patrick has a B.Sc. in Biology from Queen's University, a M.Sc. in Global Health from the Brighton and Sussex Medical School and a Ph.D. in Population Health from the University of Ottawa. His doctoral research involved the development of a mathematical model to assess the preparedness of Canadian hospitals to accommodate surges in patient demand associated with influenza. He also holds a certificate in risk-based decision making for public and population health, and teaches two courses at Carleton University: Global Health Governance and Pandemics and Infectious Diseases. Patrick lives in Ottawa with his wife and dog.

Patrick's other publications on pandemic influenza include:

- Saunders-Hastings, P., Quinn Hayes, B., Smith, R., & Krewski, D. (2017). National assessment of Canadian pandemic preparedness: employing InFluNet to identify high-risk areas for inter-wave vaccine distribution. *Infectious Disease Modelling*, *2*(3), 341–352.
- Saunders-Hastings, P., Quinn Hayes, B., Smith, R., & Krewski, D. (2017). Modelling community-control strategies to protect hospital resources during an influenza pandemic in Ottawa, Canada. *PLoS One, 12*(6), e0179315.
- Saunders-Hastings, P., Crispo, J., Sikora, L., & Krewski, D. (2017). Assessing the effectiveness of personal protective measures in reducing pandemic influenza transmission: a systematic review. *Epidemics, 20*, 1–20.

- Saunders-Hastings, P., Reisman, J., & Krewski, D. (2016). Assessing the state of knowledge regarding the effectiveness of interventions to contain pandemic influenza transmission: a systematic review and narrative synthesis. *PLoS One, 11*(12), e0168262.
- Saunders-Hastings, P. & Krewski, D. (2016). Reviewing the history of pandemic influenza: Understanding patterns of emergence and transmission. *Pathogens, 5*(4), 66.

In: Pandemics
Editor: Pavel I. Sidorov
ISBN: 978-1-53614-274-7

Chapter 4

USING SOCIAL MEDIA FOR PANDEMIC MANAGEMENT

Marjorie Greene *
Center for Naval Analyses (CNA)
Arlington, VA, US

ABSTRACT

This chapter recommends using social media to automate the ability of organizations to coordinate their activities during pandemics. It is based on an innovative approach that constructs online networks of email and text messages as they evolve in real time. Based on a unique message addressing rule that takes advantage of "emergent intelligence", the approach shows how pandemics can be managed in real time. I do this by tracking all communications in a chain of messages that are sent from person to person on a topic related to the pandemic. Then, as the community of interest grows, my approach creates a "closed network" that isolates it from the larger social network. The major benefit of this approach is that it provides feedback because it guarantees that all organizations in the network are automatically kept informed of all previous organizations that participated in the message chain. In this way,

* Corresponding author: greenem@cna.org.

I mimic the famous experiments of social psychologist Stanley Milgram, who provided the first empirical evidence of "six degrees of separation" when constructing paths via letters from person to person to achieve a goal.

Keywords: social media, closed network, emergent intelligence, biological threat, self-organizing systems, pandemic management

INTRODUCTION

Not long ago, the Center for Bio-security at the University of Pittsburgh Medical Center sponsored an article by S. S. Morse on Public Health Surveillance and Infectious Disease Detection. Dr. Morse (Morse 2012) points out that "the rise of social networking has the potential to play an increasingly important role in the future. As with digital disease detection (DDD), this revolution in communications technology promises to break down many of the barriers to reporting, but at the risk of increasing the noise level and volume of raw data and the difficulty of verifying reports…." The article suggests that the pandemic management challenge of the future will be to develop tools to effectively exploit social networks while maintaining the benefits of official reports from government authorities.

1. REFERENCE-CONNECTED SETS

I have developed (Greene 2011) a self-organizing ontology that allows the filtering of e-mail messages in such a way that obstacles created by information overload can be overcome. I tested my methodology on ProMED-mail, the largest reporting base of any health organization, and found that it works! The unique attribute of ProMED-mail is that it uses references to "track" reports of disease evolution. Messages cite references to previous messages on the same or related outbreaks. Often a message references a previous message which references a yet earlier message. I found that if all messages related to each other through their references were retrieved, the resulting "reference-connected set" of messages uniquely identified biological threats of pandemics. This is especially valuable to epidemiologists who can now quickly track the evolution of specific outbreaks for further analysis. Perhaps the greatest benefit of this classification system is that it can be generated dynamically and constructed in real time as it evolves.

2. A Pro-Active Approach

Agencies that manage pandemics may be able to pro-actively construct reference-connected sets. They would do this by sending messages to each other on specific events and keeping track of previous messages on the same event, thus creating a path from person to person that tracks the event. This ability to reference previous messages on the same event has not been automated. And it is not yet possible to easily track messages in a social network. It may therefore make sense to develop a Web-based tool that will help both civilian and military agencies exploit social networks for the detection of biological threats.

2.1. Vannevar Bush

Vannevar Bush was perhaps the first person to come up with a new way of thinking about searching for information (Bush 1945). He suggested that an individual's personal information storage and selection system could be based on direct connections between documents instead of the usual connections between index terms and documents. These direct connections were to be stored in the form of trails through the literature. Then at any future time the individual himself or one of his associates could retrieve this trail from document to document without the necessity of describing each document with a set of descriptors or tracing it down through a classification tree. Scientists have also suggested grouping scientific papers through "bibliographic coupling", and many projects have been funded to develop advanced software and algorithms for searching, filtering, and summarizing large volumes of data, imagery, and all kinds of information in an environment in which users are linked through interconnected communications networks without the benefit of pre-established criteria for arranging content.

2.2. Norbert Wiener

In his book "Cybernetics", Norbert Wiener (1965) brought the insights and techniques of many disciplines to bear on problems of communication and control. Now well established as a field of study which deals with the role of feed-back both in engineering design and in biology, cybernetics can also be applied to many of the approaches to learning and self-organizing systems that are being explored today. More recent studies have also shown that feedback loops are an essential requirement for control when decisions are made during crises. It has been shown that information flows break down with more than three decision-makers in a non-hierarchical organization, and many researchers feel that a clear command structure is still needed for control in collaborative decision making. An example of the importance of feedback loops has been found in socio-technical analyses of the SARS outbreak, where analysts have concluded that a lack of feedback explains why SARS was widely transmitted.

Professor Wiener also discusses another concept in his book that is beginning to capture the interest of a multi-disciplinary community. He points out that intercommunication of ants, in which the only means of communication appears to be the sense of smell, seems to lead to a highly standardized course of conduct in which information is conveyed. This led to his conclusion that social animals may have an active, intelligent, flexible means of communication that results in communal information that can be distinguished from the amount of information available to the individual members of the community. An example of this phenomenon, which he called "emergent behavior", is the ant routing algorithm which tells us that when an ant forages for food, it lays pheromones on a trail from source to destination.

When it arrives at its destination, it returns to the source following the same path it came from. If other ants have travelled the same path, pheromone value is higher. Similarly, if other ants have not travelled along the path, the pheromone level is lower. If every ant tries to choose the trail that has higher pheromone concentration, eventually the pheromones accumulate when multiple ants use the same path and evaporate when no ant passes. A growing number of research scientists are beginning to explore emergent behavior as an approach to the study of complex adaptive systems which are characterized by "agents" interacting with each other in dynamic, often nonlinear and surprising ways.

2.3. Stanley Milgram

Stanley Milgram was a social psychologist who performed a series of experiments in the 1960's that provided the first empirical evidence of "six degrees of separation" describing the notion that we are all just a few steps apart in the global social network. His hypothesis was that short paths can be found in "social networks" that could be used to quickly reach a target destination when an individual mails a letter to someone he or she knows on a first-name basis, with the instructions to forward it on in this way toward the target as quickly as possible. The letter eventually moved from friend to friend, with the successful letters reaching the target in a median of six steps. This kind of experiment – constructing paths through social networks to distant target individuals – has been repeated by a number of other groups in subsequent decades.

3. A National Pandemic Challenge

Techniques for understanding how to effectively exploit social behavior in managing pandemics are still in their initial stages. Does the social network have an ability to "funnel" information on pandemics without any central control? Would it be possible to combine Vannevar Bush's model of "trails of messages" with Norbert Wiener's "emergent behavior" approach to proactively construct paths through social networks to improve pandemic management? Could a dynamic information retrieval system be based on communications paths and direct connections between individual communicators rather than upon traditional technologies that mechanically or electronically select information from a store? We have an opportunity to address this next-generation research challenge, and this paper suggests the development of a tool to do this as a benefit to society and a contribution to an important pandemic management need.

3.1. Approach

Just as an ant leaves a chemical trace of its movement along a path, my simulated agent attaches traces of its previous contacts by means of "digital pheromones" to each message that it sends. I do this by ensuring that all communicators along the path are kept informed of all previous communicators in the path. Suppose, for example, that "A", "B" and "C" are three individuals in a social network. "A" starts a path reporting on a particular event by sending a message to "B". "B", in turn, decides to send a message to "C" on the same event. Thus far, this is similar to the Milgram experiment, in which a "path" was created as a letter was forwarded from friend to friend until it reached a designated "target" in the network. However, in this case, the target "emerges" from the interaction of A, B, and C. Another major difference is that I apply a simple message-addressing rule that asks each individual to "copy" all previous individuals on an event (say, in the "cc" line in an email message) when he chooses to send a message on that event. (A tool can be developed to automate this process.) A sequence of messages is thus created that is based on communications between individuals reporting on a biological threat, and this "path" represents an evolving threat. We have thus reversed the "reference-connected set" process by constructing a path in a social network that identifies threats and classifies them as they occur in real time.

3.2. A Pilot-Test

It may be possible to pilot-test a tool for pandemic management in partnership with ProMED-mail. ProMED-mail is an official program of the International Society of Infectious Diseases and the largest reporting base of any health organization. As noted above, it has a unique attribute of citing references when it reports on disease outbreaks. In this way, the evolution of an outbreak can be "tracked", and when messages related in any way through their references are retrieved, the resulting "reference-connected set" will identify a specific biological event. The tool would be designed to effectively exploit social networks in the identification of biological threats by filtering out the noise in social networks and giving authorities the ability to complement existing reports on emerging infectious diseases. The tool should be able to match the speed with which the general public is able to spread information using social media. Ultimately, the tool would have the ripple effect of providing any government agency the ability to obtain an early warning of a biological event as it evolves in real time.

3.3. Benefits

The application of "digital pheromones" that result in trails of messages related to a pandemic has several benefits in addition to giving authorities the ability to identify, analyze, and report as reliably and quickly as possible:

- The approach will help epidemiologists in their effort to trace outbreaks and to identify their origin. Laboratory tests for an outbreak's identification can be initiated more quickly.
- Because all reporters along the path are automatically kept informed of all previous reporters in the path, it achieves the important feedback loop identified by Norbert Wiener as an essential requirement for control when decisions are made during crises.
- The approach avoids the need to define an evolving pandemic which may not fit into a pre-determined classification category.
- The approach can be used as a planning tool to help in the analysis of ways in which social media can be used to provide information, thus enhancing situational awareness during a pandemic.

Conclusion

The Sunday, March 4, 2018 Outlook Section of the Washington Post noted that the Spanish flu pandemic brought new urgency to the quest to comprehend infectious diseases but that the subject is still beset by scientific challenges and popular misunderstandings. The article points out the most tenacious myths, including the myth that a pandemic on the scale of Spanish flu is unlikely today. In my opinion, we must be prepared to cope with such a pandemic in the future. There are several tools already available using social media that could and should be pilot tested.

References

Bush, V. (1945). As We May Think, *Atlantic Monthly*. 176 (1): 101-108.

Greene, M. (2011). Using Social Media to Communicate During Crises: *An Analytic Methodology,* CNA PP D0024034.A4/2REV.

Morse, S. S. (2012). *Biosecurity and Bioterrorism: Biodefense Strategy, Practice, & Science,* 10 (1): 6-16, DOI: 10.1089/bsp.2011.0088.
Wiener, N. (1965). *Cybernetics: Or Control and Communications in the Animal and Machine*. Edition 2. Paris. MIT Press. P. 212.

Biographical Sketch

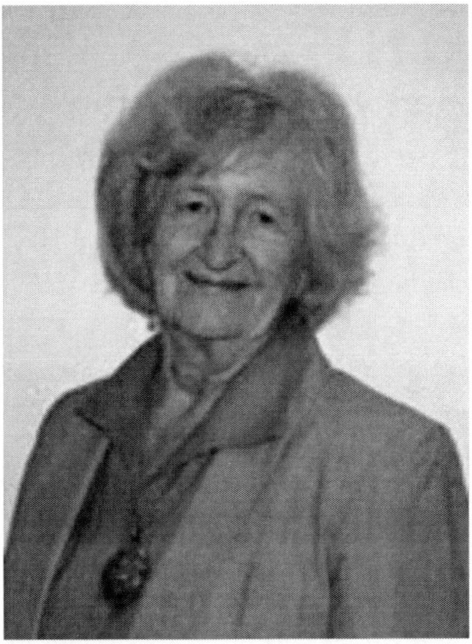

Marjorie Greene has more than 25 years' management experience in both government and commercial organizations and has recently specialized in finding S&T solutions for the U.S. Marine Corps. She has provided overall approaches to clarify mission objectives; organized, directed, and coordinated strategic planning activities; provided guidance for building operational plans and specifying measurable outcomes; and facilitated multidisciplinary projects, including: workshops, modeling technological systems for humanitarian relief, outreach to organizations to explore engineering solutions to the development of strategic S&T products, war games, and military utility assessments.

Education

Ph.D., Operations Research, Johns Hopkins University, Baltimore, MD
Course Work Completed, June, 1971
M.A., Mathematics, University of Nebraska, Lincoln, Nebraska, 1961
B.S., Mathematics, Creighton University, Omaha, Nebraska, 1955

Work History

CAN, Research Analyst, 2010 - 2013
Conducted study for ONR of S&T Solutions for the USMC Logistics Chain
Supported research on Rapid and Affordable Naval HA/DR
Developed analytic methodology for using Social Media during crises
SAIC, Senior Program Manager, 1997 - 2010
Contractor to ONR - Specified measurable outcomes to operational plans; met with Government personnel to facilitate multi-agency projects, conducted workshops, organized outreach activities.
National Y2K Information Coordination Center supporting President's Council -- responsible for relationships with Federal agencies.

Principal Investigator for Projects to Evaluate New Technologies

ANSER Senior Policy Analyst, 1995 - 1997
Responsible for Business Process Reengineering program
DHHS Independent Contractor, 1992 - 1995
Developed metrics to evaluate success of Health and Human Services initiatives
CAP/SEMA Consulting, London, England, Director, 1988 - 1992
Established new business offering IT solutions for banking industry
Harvard University Index Group, London, England, Senior Associate, 1985 - 1988

Matched technology initiatives to commercial objectives
First Chicago Corporation, Vice President, 1981 - 1985
Responsible for competitive analyses
Inter-Bank Research Organization, London, England, Senior Associate, 1977 - 1981
Coordinated planning for payment systems
American Express Company Director, 1974 - 1977
Coordinated relationships with members of the National EFT Commission
Executive Office of the President, Program Manager, 1971 - 1974
Coordinated Government telecommunications systems

Project Experience

Title: PONCE Deployment
Client: MSC
Period of Performance: 10/2013 - present
Role: Met with MSC to develop project proposal
Documented/analyzed requirements

Title: Stability and Security Operations Wargame
Client: CAPE
Period of Performance: 10/2011 - 01/2012
Role: Reviewer

Documented Observations/Issues for Program Evaluation

Title: Gaming Airpower in Counter-Insurgency and Irregular Warfare Campaign
Client: OSD
Period of Performance: 01/2012
Role: Reviewer
Documented observations/issues for program evaluation

Title: S&T for Communications and Persuasion Overseas: Gap Analysis and Survey
Client: RRTO, DASD
Period of Performance: 2011 - 2012
Role: Reviewer
Noted implications of mobile devices that are becoming the primary means of accessing information and communications devices like the Internet

Title: S&T Solutions for the USMC Logistics Chain
Client: ONR
Period of Performance: 2010 - 2012
Role: Project Director
Initiated study, discussed/refined study issues with sponsor, identified requirements, identified external support requirements, conducted interviews, coordinated study results

Title: Information Flows During the Domrep Crisis
Client: CNO
Period of Performance: 1964 - 1967
Role: Project Director
Published several studies as an analyst with OEG in a field assignment at the Pentagon

Expertise/Keywords

C4ISR, Digital Disease Detection, Social Networking, Operations Analysis, Integration of Military-Civilian Operations During Crises

Publications and Reports

PHALANX Magazine, Sept 2013 Issue

CNA PP D0024034.A4/2REV, July 2011
CME D0026056.A1/Final, Oct 2011
Proceedings of SPIE Defense Security & Sensing, Vol.7666, 2010
NSF White Paper, 2010
SPIE Proceedings, 2011
MORS Symposium Presentations, 2009, 2010, 2011, 2012
ASNE Journal, 2010
PHALANX, Sept 2009
IEEE Technology and Society Magazine, Fall, 1997

Professional Associations

Military Operations Research Society -- Trustee
IEEE - Medical Technology Policy Committee, Bioterrorism Working Group
The Military Conflict Institute (TMCI)
American Society of Naval Engineers

Clearance Level

Top Secret, 2001 - 2018

Marjorie Greene was the first female analyst to work at CNA, arriving after earning her master's degree in mathematics and spending two years in the very first cohort of Peace Corps volunteers. A field assignment at sea was still out of the question in that era, so Marjorie was assigned to the CNO Flag Plot in the Pentagon to analyze command-and-control operations during crises. Though she left CNA after a few years when she and her husband moved to London, she retained such fond memories that after a long career with other organizations, she returned in 2010 as a part-time analyst and remains a part of CNA today.

In: Pandemics
Editor: Pavel I. Sidorov
ISBN: 978-1-53614-274-7

Chapter 5

PANDEMIC OF ARCTIC SUICIDALITY

Yury Sumarokov**, *MD, PhD
International School of Public Health,
Northern State Medical University, Arkhangelsk, Russia

ABSTRACT

This is a study of suicides in the Russian Arctic with the focus on the Nenets Autonomous Okrug (NAO), a region with a large proportion of indigenous people.

As a starting point, we conducted a retrospective population-based mortality study of suicides in the NAO, using data from the autopsy reports of suicide victims in the region in 2002-2012. Socio-demographic data were obtained from passports and medical records, and then linked to the total population data from the 2002 and 2010 censuses. Suicide rates for indigenous Nenets and non-indigenous population were calculated according to different socio-demographic characteristics, and corresponding relative risks for these two populations were compared. Variations in suicide methods, seasonal variations, and variations in the day of the week suicides occurred in the NAO were compared with national data from the Russian Federal Statistics Service (Rosstat).

* Corresponding author: sioury@mail.ru.

Forensic data on the blood alcohol content in suicide cases from the NAO were compared with the data from the neighboring Arkhangelsk Oblast.

Suicide rates in the NAO were higher than corresponding national figures. Suicide rates were higher among the indigenous Nenets than the non-indigenous population, and were associated with different socio-demographic characteristics. We showed different relative frequencies of suicide by hanging, cutting, and firearm, as well as differences in suicide occurrence by month and day of the week in the NAO when compared with Russia as a whole. Alcohol may be an essential risk factor for suicide among the Arctic indigenous people.

The study results and conclusions may be useful to create suicide prevention programs that are targeted to different population groups in the Russian Arctic. The special emphasis should be done by the community based suicide prevention activities.

Keywords: suicidal pandemic, indigenous people, suicide methods, alcohol

INTRODUCTION

Suicide is a significant public health problem in all cultures and all societies (WHO 2018). Indeed, suicide represents 1.4% of the Global Burden of Disease and its economic costs are in the billions of dollars. Over the past 50 years, the number of suicides worldwide increased by approximately 60%. Almost one million fatalities every year are attributed to suicide, and in most European countries, the annual number of suicides is larger than that of traffic fatalities. The World Health Organization (WHO) has recognized the seriousness of suicide as a public health problem and has begun a global initiative for the prevention of suicide (WHO 2014).

Among countries that maintain registers on suicide, the highest rates are found in Eastern Europe and the lowest are found mostly in Latin America, in Muslim countries, and in a few of the Asian countries. However, there are few such registers in African countries (last two years the number is growing fast). Although no reliable data is available on attempted suicides, this number is estimated to be 10-20 times higher than that of completed suicides, resulting in injury, hospitalization, emotional and mental trauma. Suicide rates tend to increase with the age, but the WHO has recognized an alarming worldwide increase in suicidal behaviors among the age group of 15 to 25 years. Estimates suggest that fatalities among all age groups could rise to 1.5 million by 2020 (WHO 2018).

1. Suicide in the Indigenous Populations

A study in 1979 by Grove and Lynge (Grove, Lynge 1979) showed that suicide rates in the indigenous Inuit population in Greenland increased four-fold during the 1970s. The authors pointed to several factors, including alcohol consumption, that were associated both with the suicide and the social and cultural evolution of the Inuit society. Various studies have also reported high suicide rates among indigenous Inuit populations from the Hudson Bay (Kirmayer et al. 2000) and the Canadian Northwestern Territories (Young et al. 1992). Studies from Northern Norway showed there were more suicides among the indigenous Sami than the Norwegian general population (Silviken et al. 2006; Silviken 2009). Studies from other indigenous populations, including Aboriginal communities in Australia (Tatz 2001; Stevenson et al. 1998; De Leo et al. 2012), Native Americans in the United States (Tatz 2001; Middlebrook et al. 2001; Mock et al. 1996), the Maoris in New Zealand (Beautrais 2003), and Inuits in Greenland [3], have also shown high suicide rates. In Greenland (Grove, Lynge 1979), Canada (Chachamovich et al. 2015), Norway (Silviken 2009), Australia (Tatz 2001; Measey et al. 2006), and Brazil (Souza, Orellana 2012; Orellana et al. 2016), high suicide risk clusters were found to coincide with the territorial distribution of indigenous populations. Suicide rates in indigenous populations tend to be high, and violent suicide methods are common, especially among young males (Silviken et al. 2006; Silviken 2009; Hunter, Harvey 2002). Suicide among the indigenous people has no borders. We even can define this very common alarming health situation among the indigenous people as "suicidal pandemics." "Top-5" of the Arctic Indigenous territories by suicide rates is represented by Greenland, Nunavut (Canada), Nenets Autonomous Okrug (NAO), Chukotka (Russia), and Alaska (US).

Table 1. Cultural values of indigenous and non-indigenous peoples (Mulvad 2015)

Indigenous	Western (Non-Indigenous)
Harmony with nature	Domination of nature
Soul and body united	Soul and body are divided
Feelings are important	Feelings must be rationalized
Education from elders	Education from professionals
Material wealth is shared	Material wealth is hoarded and consumed
Behavior is cooperative	Behavior is competitive
Leaders serve the people	People serve the leaders
To be > to have	To have > to be

G. Mulvad (Mulvad 2015) concluded that indigenous peoples use multifactorial processes to define and understand the circumstances of their life, rather than taking a problem-specific approach. Many behavioral differences between indigenous and non-indigenous populations are based on their different cultural values (Table 1), and any damage to or pressure on the cultural values of indigenous peoples may lead to an increase in depression, violence, addiction problems, and suicides.

In the Russian Federation, indigenous nations are stated according to Federal Law. There are about 40 indigenous groups that reside in the Russian Arctic, Siberia, and the Russian Far East (Kryazhkov 2014). A governmental decree officially defines their status as "Indigenous small-numbered people of the North." In the Russian Arctic, almost half of these ethnic groups coexist. Some of them are rather big, like the Nenets, the Khanty, the Mansi, the Nanai, the Chukchi, and the Evenks, with population between 10,000 and 45,000. Others have less than 1000 people, like the Aleuts, the Nganasanes, the Oroks, the Chuvans, etc. Their histories share common factors of assimilation, i.e., a loss of traditional lifestyles, occupations, and ethnic identity (Polozhy 2000).

2. The History of Suicide in the Russian Arctic

Our knowledge of the history of suicide in the Russian Arctic is based on ethnographic studies that started in the 18th century. Historical studies of suicide traditions show that the Nenets and Chukchi had a custom of free-will (voluntary) self-inflicted death and self-inflicted death out of revenge in the middle of the 19th century (Zelenin 2004). Russian ethnographer Kushelevsky said that such deaths could be explained by a fear of punishment and considered them as a "sacrifice to the gods." Interestingly, in the case of such sacrifice, hanging ("strangling") was the preferred suicide method. Indeed, it was believed that disease demons could emerge from the body at the time of death, but that if hanging was used, the noose around the neck would keep any such demons from escaping. Ethnographers found several different suicide patterns and suicide traditions among indigenous people in Russia (Zelenin 2004):

- A custom of free-will (voluntary) self-inflicted death among the Chukchi and Nenets;
- A custom of voluntary death in the Chukchi called "battle with spirit(s)" (Lottery 1765; Bogoraz 1934);
- Suicide due to an inability to resist a disease (Chukchi, Nenets);
- The "Taedium vitae" phenomena (Bogoraz 1916, 1934);
- The tradition of assisted suicide by hanging in the Chukchi (Bogoraz);
- Family suicides that have been described in Eastern Siberia (Kostrov 1844);
- Suicide due to the belief that natural death was a shame in the Chukchi (Avgustinovich 1878);

- Suicide due to a belief that natural death does not exist (Koty 1933);
- Suicide as a survival strategy for families when the weak, old, and sick create problems (Bukharov 1883);
- Suicide in expectation of a better life after death in the Nenets (Kushelevsky 1868).

Ethnographic sources from the 19th century say that Russian merchants played the most important role in the formation of the drinking habits of the Nenets, who have the highest level of alcohol consumption in Northwestern Russia (Saveliev 1852). One source described how merchants from Mezen exchanged vodka for important staple items, like furs, meat, and other products with the Kolguev Nenets. All men, women, and at times even children, were drunk, and this drunkenness was often accompanied by violence, homicides, and suicides (Golovanov 2002).

When the Mezen merchants left Kolguev Island due to reindeer deaths (a result of regular tundra icing), reindeer herders from the island were hired by locals from the Nenets village of Oksino, and the situation changed radically. The reindeer herders of the Sumarokov family from Oksino banned the delivery and use of vodka on Kolguev Island. They supplied the island with all the necessary goods and did not allow other merchants into the area, fearing that the locals would fall into drunkenness. This may be the first case of intervention and prevention of alcohol abuse among the indigenous people in Russian history.

After the Russian revolution and the civil war in 1917-1920, alcohol abuse in the region worsened again, as did the preservation of the traditional way of life of the indigenous people. The supply of vodka to local residents was organized rather well. In 1919, local reindeer herder Nikita Ardeev noted, "The "Reds" [new "Bolshevik" power] brought so much alcohol to the island that the locals will not be able to drink it all until the end of next spring" (Golovanov 2002). In 1929, new regulations forced private and family reindeer operations to merge into collective farms, and the final blow to the traditional life of the Nenets people came when intensive oil extraction began in the 1980s and 1990s. After this, the lifestyle of the indigenous communities in the Russian Arctic changed dramatically. Their socioeconomic status was suppressed by the invasion of state and private mining companies, and the balance of ethnicity and nature was broken. The environmental changes, along with an undeveloped infrastructure, affected lifestyle, livelihood, culture, and physical and mental health and well-being (MacDonald et al. 2013). In the 1990s, the introduction of new economic rules finally destroyed the cultural values of the indigenous peoples of this region and increased the risk of social deprivation, stress-related mental disorders, depression, addiction, and suicidal behavior.

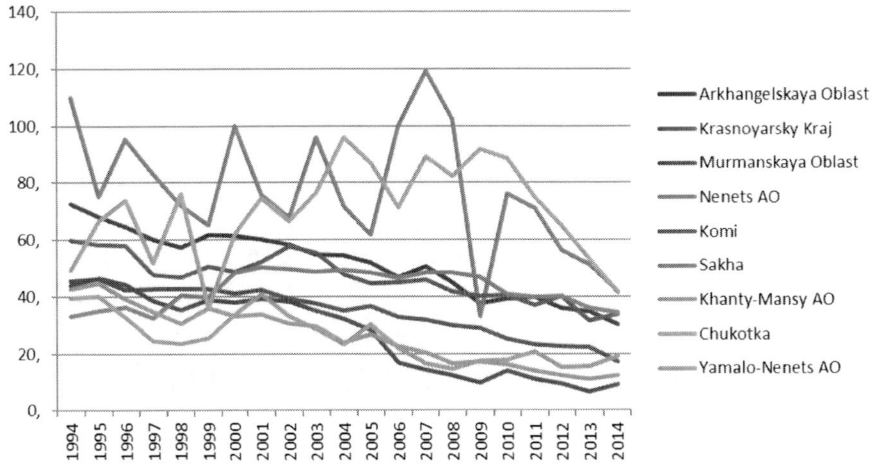

Figure 1. Suicide rates in the Russian Arctic (per 100,000 population), 1994-2014 Russian Federal Statistics Service (Rosstat) (AO: Autonomous Okrug).

Nowadays, suicide rates in the Russian Arctic (Figure 1) demonstrate the differences between the populations, lifestyles, and many other factors.

The territories with a higher proportion of indigenous people (NAO, Chukotka) have higher suicide rates (Table 2).

Table 2. Average suicide rates (per 100,000) for 1994-2014 and the proportions of indigenous people in the Russian Arctic by region. (AO: Autonomous Okrug)

Region of Russian Arctic	Average suicide rate 1994 – 2014	Proportion of indigenous population (%), Census, 2010
NAO	77.0	17.8
Chukotka	63.1	32.8
Taymyr	50.1	24.8
Yakutia	40.1	3.8
Arkhangelsk Oblast	35.6	0.7
Murmansk oblast	26.9	0.2
Yamal-Nenets AO	26.2	9.8

3. Risk and Protective Factors

There have been many studies on the risk factors for suicide in indigenous populations. Most of the risk factors are common to many different population groups, and we can assume that some of these risk factors also exist in the Nenets society. Based on the existing evidence, we propose that the risk factors for suicide in indigenous populations are subject to several levels of influence (Kirmayer et al. 1996; Inuit Tapiriit Kantanami 2016):

1. National and regional-level influence: historical trauma, impact of collectivization and industrialization, forced relocation, and settlement.
2. Community-level influence: socioeconomic inequality and lack of access to health services.
3. Family-level influence: family history of suicide, intergenerational trauma, domestic violence, and boarding schools.

4. Personality-level influence: depression, substance abuse, mental disorders, history of self-harm, acute stress, hopelessness, and isolation.
5. Conditional-level influence: easy access to the most violent means of suicide (firearms, ropes, knives) and intoxication due to alcohol or drug use.

Protective factors for suicide in indigenous populations are subject to the same influences (Inuit Tapiriit Kantanami 2016):

1. National- and regional-level influence: cultural continuity and sustainability based on language, culture, and history.
2. Community-level influence: economic, social, educational, and health equity.
3. Family-level influence: supportive family with traditional life and native language environment.
4. Personality-level influence: access to ethnicity-specific mental health, social and emotional development, coping with acute stress, high level of resilience, and religious factors.
5. Conditional-level influence: restricted access to alcohol and drugs, alcohol and drug policy measures.

There is evidence that frequency of church attendance is associated with a decreased risk of attempted suicide among the Inuit. The Nenets religious culture is a mixture of traditional spirituality and Orthodox Christianity, which is probably why religion is not a crucial protective factor for suicide among the Nenets.

4. Study

During the last few years we were conducting a retrospective, population-based mortality study of suicides in the NAO, using data from the autopsy reports of suicide victims in the region in 2002-2012. To our knowledge, that was the first study investigating the problem of suicide in the indigenous and non-indigenous populations of the Russian Arctic. Our study aim was to assess suicide rates in the indigenous and non-indigenous populations of the NAO, as well as the socio-demographic characteristics, differences in suicide methods, seasonal variations, and the potential role of alcohol in suicides in these two populations.

The aims of our study were:

1. To describe the suicide rates among the indigenous and the non-indigenous populations of the NAO in 2002-2012 and to define the socio-demographic characteristics associated with suicide in each of these populations;
2. To investigate variations in suicide rates, suicide methods, and suicide occurrence by month and day of the week among the indigenous and non-indigenous populations of the NAO and to compare the findings from NAO with national Russian statistics;
3. To investigate the potential role of alcohol and alcohol consumption on suicides in the NAO in 2002-2012 and to compare NAO data with corresponding data from Arkhangelsk Oblast (AO) for the same period.

This study does not intend to describe cultural, sociological and anthropological aspects of suicides in NAO.

We collected data on suicides that occurred in 2002-2012 in the NAO and the AO. We also obtained National data on suicides from the Russian Federation (2002-2012).

For suicides occurring during the study period in the NAO (N=252), we had data on age, ethnic group, sex, area of residence, employment status, education level, marital status, suicide method, date, month, and day of the week suicide occurred, presence of alcohol in the blood, BAC, and alcohol sales. Data on the general population of the NAO, including population size, population distribution by ethnic group, and other considered socio-demographic characteristics (sex, urban/rural residence, occupation, education level, and marital status) were obtained from the

Official Russian Censuses of 2002 and 2010. No other socio-demographic data were available on the NAO population between or after these two censuses.

For suicides occurring during the study period in the AO (N=1185), we had data on presence of alcohol in the blood, BAC, age, sex, suicide method, and alcohol sales, which were collected from the forensic records of the Arkhangelsk Bureau of Forensic Medical Expertise.

Data on suicides that occurred in the Russian Federation during the study period (N = 571,162) were obtained from the Russian Federal Statistics Service (Rosstat), using anonymous micro-data on all deaths from external causes recorded in the National Mortality Database in 2002-2012, and disaggregated by sex, suicide method, and month and day of the week suicide occurred.

The person-year (PY) approach was used to estimate suicide rates for the Nenets population and the non-indigenous population, as well as according to the considered socio-demographic characteristics within these populations. No information on history of self-harm or attempted suicide was available for the cases of suicide in the present study. For these reasons the denominators in our calculations of suicide rates were estimates rather than true numbers. The number of PY of risk in each population was computed as the average population for each ethnic group in the 2002 and 2010 censuses multiplied by 11 (number of years of observation). Suicide rates were calculated as the number of suicides per 100,000 PY. Relative risk estimates were calculated as ratios of suicide rates in analogue socio-demographic subgroups of the Nenets population and the non-indigenous population.

Data were presented as absolute numbers and proportions. The Chi-square test and Fisher's exact test were used to calculate the differences in categorical variables between the studied groups. To test whether the distribution of suicides in the studied groups was equal on the time axes (months of the year and days of the week), the observed distribution of suicides was compared with a hypothesized equal distribution by the Chi-square goodness of fit test. Microsoft Excel and IBM SPSS Statistics v.21.0 were used for data storage and analyses.

The study was approved on 23 June 2010 by the Ethical Committee of the Northern State Medical University, Arkhangelsk, Russia. None of the data variables accessed for the purposes of this study by non-employees of the health centers and forensic bureau could be used for personal identification.

5. RESULTS

The most relevant findings from the study are:

The suicide rate in the indigenous Nenets population of the NAO is higher than in the non-indigenous population in the region, and higher than the national average in Russia. The most vulnerable age groups were 20-29 years in men and 30-39 years in women. Single or divorced individuals also showed a higher risk (Sumarokov et al. 2014).

Hanging was the most common suicide method in females, whereas men more frequently used firearms and cutting. April was the month with the highest occurrence of suicide, and Friday was the weekday with the highest suicide incidence (Sumarokov et al. 2015).

Alcohol was found in the blood of three-quarters of male suicide cases and more than four-fifths of female suicide cases in the NAO, compared with 59.3% and 46% in the AO, respectively. Corresponding figures for the indigenous population of the NAO were even higher, with 78.3% in males and 92.3% in females. The highest occurrence of alcohol in the blood was found in females who committed suicide by hanging and in males using knives or firearms (Sumarokov et al. 2016).

Here, the NAO could be used as an example of an Arctic region with a high indigenous population. How could this information be applied in prevention programs for the indigenous population in the NAO?

First, the indigenous population needs to get information about the results of this study. This must take place in meetings with local health authorities and leaders of the indigenous population. It is crucial to focus on the indigenous lifestyle and activities in the seasons when most suicides take place, and to identify potential stress factors that may increase the risk of suicide. A variety of hypotheses should be discussed and tested, including the change in physiology and hormonal activity, darkness – lightness problems, and change in lifestyle connected with seasonal activity, which characterizes the life of indigenous peoples. Emphasis should be put on the age groups with the highest risk, and on the single and divorced individuals within these age groups.

CONCLUSION

Old superstitions and beliefs may represent an extra risk for females who commit suicide by hanging. Firm and convincing information on this item from health authorities is essential if these old beliefs are to be ruled out as an important act to honor the gods.

Alcohol seems to play an important role in suicides among indigenous peoples, as has been seen in similar populations in other countries. Lawmakers and local authorities must be convinced that measures need to be taken in order to reduce alcohol intake in the population (Public Chamber of Russian Federation 2009). Accessibility to and prices of alcohol are essential in this connection, and some restrictions have already been introduced in the NAO. In addition to accessibility and prices, opening hours, an age-limit for buying liquor, restricted opening hours before holidays and long weekends, not selling to drunk people, and eventual quota regulations should be considered (Public Chamber of Russian Federation 2009).

This is the first study of suicides among the indigenous people of the Russian Arctic, and there is a strong motivation to continue our research. Further studies of suicide among the Nenets and other Arctic indigenous groups are needed. These studies should also give us more information on attempted suicide among the Nenets, and provide data on the frequency, severity, and duration of suicidal thoughts. These studies should combine different approaches, including quantitative and qualitative methods, and analyze environmental, genetic, and psychological factors that influence suicidal behavior among the Nenets. For this large-scale surveys will be necessary (Nock et al. 2012).

To increase the knowledge on the situation that existed before suicide, a psychological autopsy could be applied: a forensic psychologist or a skilled clinical psychologist would interview the family, friends, or colleagues of suicide victims. The resultant information on the status of deceased individuals before they took their life may be of use for preventive measures.

These measures, especially performed on the community level, will decrease the risks of developing suicidal pandemics among the indigenous people. Most of the best examples of these strategies are well investigated in Australia, Canada and US.

The last initiative of Arctic Council (2015-2017), known as “Reducing the Incidence of Suicide in Indigenous Groups – Strengths United through Networks” (RISING SUN) has created a common set of community-based outcomes for use in evaluating suicide prevention interventions across the Arctic States (Reducing the Incidence of Suicide in Indigenous Groups 2018). The new toolkit was developed by consensus between the different groups involved in the process of developing including indigenous leaders, health workers, researchers, politicians, etc. These outcomes and their corresponding measures will support the health workers to enhance their community based services. The policy makers can use the toolkit for evaluation of interventions, and for recognition of different challenges to implementation. Strong political support and common efforts of all the Arctic states will help to win in the struggle with indigenous suicidal pandemics in the Arctic.

REFERENCES

Beautrais, A. (2003). Suicide in New Zealand I: time trends and epidemiology. *N Z Med J*. 116(1175):U460.

Chachamovich, E., Kirmayer, L. J., Haggarty, J. M., Cargo, M., McCormick, R., Turecki, G. (2015). Suicide among Inuit: Results from a Large, Epidemiologically Representative Follow-Back Study in Nunavut. *Can J Psychiatry*. 60(6):268-75.

De Leo, D., Milner, A., Sveticic, J. (2012). Mental disorders and communication of intent to die in indigenous suicide cases, Queensland, Australia. *Suicide Life-Threat*. 42(2):136-46.

Golovanov, V. (2002). *Ostrov ili opravdanie bessmyslennyh puteshestvij [Island or justification of senseless journeys]*. Moscow. Vagrius. [in Russian].

Grove, O., Lynge, J. (1979). Suicide and attempted suicide in Greenland. A controlled study in Nuuk (Godthaab). *Acta Psychiatr Scand*. 60(4):375-91.

Hunter, E., Harvey, D. (2002). Indigenous suicide in Australia, New Zealand, Canada, and the United States. *Emerg Med*. 14(1):14-23.

Inuit Tapiriit Kantanami (2016). National Strategy to prevent suicide among Canada's Inuit. Ottawa. 12.

Kirmayer, L. J., Brass, G. M., Tait, C. L. (2000). The mental health of Aboriginal peoples: transformations of identity and community. *Can J Psychiatry*. 45(7):607-16.

Kirmayer, L. J., Malus, M., Boothroyd, L. J. (1996). Suicide attempts among Inuit youth: a community survey of prevalence and risk factors. *Acta Psychiatr Scand*. 94(1):8-17.

Kryazhkov, V. (2014). Development of Russian legislation on Northern Indigenous Peoples. *Arctic Review on Law and Politics*. 4(2); 140-55.

MacDonald, J. P., Ford, J. D., Willox, A. C., Ross, N. A. (2013). A review of protective factors and causal mechanisms that enhance the mental health of Indigenous Circumpolar youth. *Int J Circumpol Heal*. 72:21775.

Measey, M. A., Li, S. Q., Parker, R., Wang, Z. (2006). Suicide in the Northern Territory, 1981-2002. *Med J Aust*. 185(6):315-19.

Middlebrook, D. L., LeMaster, P. L., Beals, J., Novins, D. K., Manson, S. M. (2001). Suicide prevention in American Indian and Alaska Native communities: a critical review of programs. *Suicide Life-Threat*. 31 Suppl:132-49.

Mock, C. N., Grossman, D. C., Mulder, D., Stewart, C., Koepsell, T. S. (1996). Health care utilization as a marker for suicidal behavior on an American Indian Reservation. *J Gen Int Med.* 11(9):519-24.

Mulvad, G. (2015). Regional Perspectives on Mental Wellness Interventions in Various Settings. *Circumpolar Mental Wellness Symposium*. Igualuit, Canada.

Nock, M., Borges, G., Ono, Y. (2012). *Suicide: Global Perspectives from the WHO World Mental Health Surveys.* Cambridge University Press.

Orellana, J. D., Balieiro, A. A., Fonseca, F. R., Basta, P. C., Souza, M. L. (2016). Spatial-temporal trends and risk of suicide in Central Brazil: an ecological study contrasting indigenous and non-indigenous populations. *Rev Bras Psiquiatr*. 38(3):222-30.

Polozhy, B. (2000). Ethnocultural peculiarities of suicide prevalence in Russia. *Eur Psychiat.* 15, Supplement 2(0):274-75.

Public Chamber of Russian Federation (2009). *Alcohol in the Russian Federation: socio-economic impacts and countermeasures*. Moscow.

Reducing the Incidence of Suicide in Indigenous Groups – Strengths United through Networks (RISING SUN) [https://www.nimh.nih.gov/about/organization/gmh/risingsun/index.shtml]. Accessed 5 March 2018.

Saveliev, A. (1852). *Die Insel Kolguev.* Archiv fur Wissenschaftlige Kunde von Russland. [*The Island Kolguev*. Archive for Wissenschaftlige customer of Russia]. X 302-18. [in German].

Silviken, A. (2009). Prevalence of suicidal behaviour among indigenous Sami in Northern Norway. *Int J Circumpol Heal*. 68:204-11.

Silviken, A., Halvordsen, T., Kvernmo, S. (2006). Suicide among Indigenous Sami in Arctic Norway 1970-1998. *Eur J Epidemiol.* 21:707-13.

Souza, M. L., Orellana, J. D. (2012). Suicide among the indigenous people in Brazil: a hidden public health issue. *Rev Bras Psiquiatr*. 34(4):489-92.

Stevenson, M. R., Wallace, L. J., Harrison, J., Moller, J., Smith, R. J. (1998). At risk in two worlds: injury mortality among indigenous people in the US and Australia, 1990-92. *Aust N Z J Public Health.* 22(6):641-44.

Suicide huge but preventable public health problem, says *WHO* [http://www.who.int/mediacentre/news/releases/2004/pr61/en/]. Accessed 16 February 2018.

Sumarokov, Y. A., Brenn, T., Kudryavtsev, A. V., Nilssen, O. (2014). Suicides in the indigenous and non-indigenous populations in the Nenets Autonomous Okrug, Northwestern Russia, and associated socio-demographic characteristics. *Int J Circumpolar Health.* 73:24308.

Sumarokov, Y. A., Brenn, T., Kudryavtsev, A. V., Nilssen, O. (2015). Variations in suicide method and in suicide occurrence by season and day of the week in Russia and the Nenets Autonomous Okrug, Northwestern Russia: a retrospective population-based mortality study. *BMC Psychiatry*. 15:224.

Sumarokov, Y. A., Brenn, T., Kudryavtsev, A. V., Sidorenkov, O., Nilssen, O. (2016). Alcohol and suicides in the Nenets Autonomous Okrug and Arkhangelsk Oblast, *Russia. Int J Circumpolar Health.* 75:30965.

Tatz, C. (2001). Confronting Australian genocide. *Aborig Hist*. 25:16-36.

World Health Organization (2014). Preventing suicide: a global imperative. Geneva. *World Health Organization*. 92.

Young, T. K., Moffatt, M. E., O'Neill, J. D. (1992). An epidemiological perspective of injuries in the Northwest Territories. *Arctic Med Res*. 51 Suppl 7:27-36.

Zelenin, D. (2004). *Izbrannye trudy: Stat'i po duhovnoj kul'ture 1934-1954 [Selected writings: papers on spiritual culture. 1934-1954]*, Moscow: Indrik. [in Russian].

Biographical Sketch

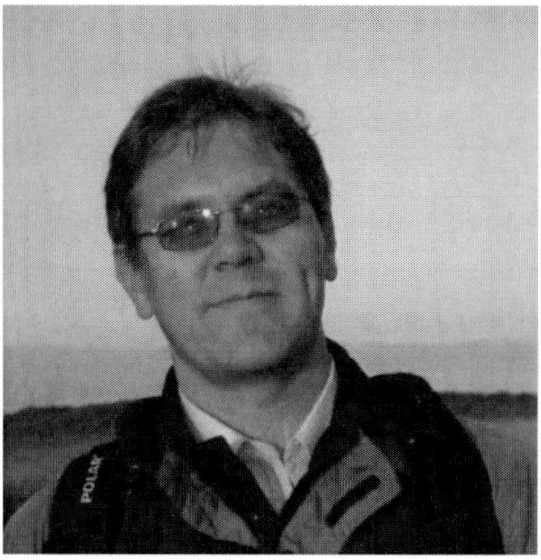

Yury Sumarokov is the Head of the Department of International cooperation at Northern State Medical University (Arkhangelsk, Russia).

Yury Sumarokov graduated MD from the Arkhangelsk State Medical Institute (Arkhangelsk, Russia) in 1983 and PhD from UiT- The Arctic University of Norway (Tromsø, Norway) in 2016. He worked as rural practitioner in Nyandoma district of Arkhangelsk oblast for 15 years.

He was then Chief Physician of Regional Psychiatry Hospital #1 (the biggest mental clinic in the North of Russia with 750 beds). During 2001-2003, he organized the Medical Information and Analytics Center in Arkhangelsk. During the same period, Yury was involved as an expert of the EU TACIS project in the areas of health management, prevention and primary health care. Since 2003 Yury has worked at the Northern State Medical University and coordinated the international co-operation program. Yury Sumarokov is representing NSMU in the University of Arctic since 2004.

He became a director of Arkhangelsk International School of Public Health (ISPHA) at the first stage of the project in 2006 – 2008. He is involved in ISPHA as co-teacher of MPH – training module "Mental Health and addictive behavior." His major research interest focused on the problem of suicides among the indigenous and non-indigenous populations of Russian North. Since 2010, he was doing research in cooperation with the Department of Community Medicine at UiT-The Arctic University of Norway. This study is the result of a long-term cooperation between the University of Tromsø (UiT) - The Arctic University of Norway and the Northern State Medical University.

Yury pointed: "I want to thank all my Northern ancestors for being my historical touchstones and for all my childhood memories, from my grandfather, Alexander Khatanzeyskiy, to all the reindeer herders of the Nenets tundra and Northern Ural. Let me also thank my father, Alexander Sumarokov, for showing me the historical significance of the local customs and regions, as well as the importance of showing respect to the local people of these regions."

In 2007 Yury met Andrey Apitsyn, Chief of the Department of Health of the Nenets Autonomous Okrug (NAO). This was at a time when Yury and his colleagues were promoting public health education in different regions of Northwestern Russia. Sumarokov came there as a teacher of a module called "Mental health and addictive behavior." He was recruiting students for our Master's program in public health at the newly-opened International School of Public Health in Arkhangelsk, for which he was responsible. Dr Apitsyn specifically emphasized suicide and alcohol abuse as the main contributors to mental health problems in the NAO, especially in the indigenous population. During this conversation, Yury was motivated to look into this problem to see if it was suitable for the deepest research.

"From my point of view, a study of this type should explain the reasons for suicides in the NAO, define the high-risk groups, and come up with possible suggestions for prevention. In 2008, after repeated meetings with several representatives of the health sector, we started to prepare a more detailed research plan, and in 2010 we signed an Agreement of Co-operation with local health authorities. The project was called "Suicide in the Nenets Autonomous Okrug, Russia" (Yury Sumarokov).

This was the first study of suicides among the indigenous people of the Russian Arctic, and there was a strong motivation to continue our research. Further studies of suicidal pandemics among the Nenets and other Arctic indigenous groups are needed. These studies should also give us more information on attempted suicide among the Arctic Indigenous people, and provide data on the frequency, severity, and duration of suicidal thoughts. These studies should combine different approaches, including quantitative and qualitative methods, and analyze environmental, genetic, and psychological factors that influence pandemic of Arctic suicidality.

In: Pandemics
Editor: Pavel I. Sidorov
ISBN: 978-1-53614-274-7

Chapter 6

PSYCHIC TRAUMATIZATION OF CHILDHOOD AS A GLOBAL PREDICTOR OF THE EPIGENETIC PANDEMIC OF MENTAL IMMUNODEFICIENCY

Pavel I. Sidorov*[*], *MD, PhD
Institute of Mental Medicine, Northern State Medical University, Arkhangelsk, Russia

ABSTRACT

The established feature of the modern world is a steady growth on the prevalence of all the major psychiatric disorders. The global predictor of this trend is the psychic traumatization of childhood and chronic psychosocial stress, triggering cumulative mechanisms of neuroepigenetic and epidemic development of mental immunodeficiency.

The task of the study is to describe the dynamics of the syndrome of mental immunodeficiency (SMID) in the early psychic traumatization of children. Mental immunity (MI) is a multimodal interface of

[*] Corresponding author: pavelsidorov13@gmail.com.

consciousness and biopsychosociospiritual identity matrix as the basis for the security of the individual and society. The pathogenetic basis of the SMID is epigenetic accumulation in many generations of functional (reversible and dynamic) MI disorders that predetermine the change in the level and quality of mental health.

In the development of an epigenetic pandemic of traumatogenic mental immunodeficiency, six fractals are identified: 1) traumatogenic family; 2) pre-traumatic diathesis; 3) acute psychic trauma; 4) full-scale clinical picture; 5) chronization; 6) outcome. The main clinical manifestations of MI dysfunctions as a multimodal interface between identity and consciousness of an individual and habitat are described and systematized. Thus, the "missing link" between epigenetic pathogenesis and clinical pathoplasty of mental disorders is found. Multidisciplinary preventive-corrective and treatment-rehabilitation protocols and programs on the technological platform of mental medicine are proposed. The expression of Nobel laureate Peter Medawar, which became a textbook: "*Genetics* proposes, *epigenetics* disposes", is appropriate to be supplemented by the mission of mental medicine, which embodies and implements project models of quality and style, the image and meaning of life in the adaptive neuroengineering and self-management of consciousness and health.

Keywords: neuroepigenetics, mental medicine, mental immunity, pandemic of mental immunodeficiency, early trauma, existential stress, "traumatogenic epigenome", multimodal interface of consciousness, biopsychosociospiritual identity matrix

INTRODUCTION

The feature of the modern world is a steady increase in the prevalence of all major mental and psychosomatic disorders. The global predictor of this trend is in many ways the psychic traumatization of childhood and chronic existential stress. They trigger transgenerational and cumulative mechanisms of epigenetic development of the pandemic of mental immunodeficiency (PMID). The task of the study is to describe and systematize epigenetic dysfunctions of MI, clinically manifested by the SMID and triggering epidemiological cascade: mental epidemic - destructive mental epidemic - pandemic of mental immunodeficiency. Early stress has both acute and long-term effects on epigenetic labels in the brain, which are the interface of MI, affecting cognitive functions and behavior, the risk of suicide and injurious acts or civil wrongdoing, dependent and psychic disorders throughout the life of today's and tomorrow's generations. SMID is clinically represented by a variety of borderline identity disorders. The pathogenetic basis of the SMID is the epigenetic accumulation of functional (reversible and dynamic) disturbances in the MI as a multimodal interface of consciousness and a biopsychosociospiritual identity matrix and the basis of security of the individual and society.

The MI is in many respects a standard placeholder, denoting the missing or indeterminate parameter or operator in the network of the relationship between identity and behavior genome and epigenome. Functional family diagnostics and screening in mental medicine (MM) make it possible to focus clinical research on the entire accessible generational line: great-grandchildren – grandchildren – children – parents – grandparents – great-grandparents. This makes it possible to assess and predict latent genetic and epigenetic predictors by calculating probabilistic scenarios and trajectories of development of destinies. Our long-term studies of the early psychic traumatization of childhood have shown the multivariance of changes in MI and biopsychosociospiritual characteristics of the "traumatogenic family", depending on the severity and duration of transgenerational stress burden. The clinical features of new generations of the "traumatogenic epigenome" depended significantly on external conditions: the same behavioral models (which are constant for humanity) gave completely opposite effects in different social environments. That is why only the synergetic biopsychosociospiritual methodology of MM allows designing effective integrative programs for the protection of public health.

1. Synergetic Biopsychosociospiritual Methodology of Mental Medicine

Synergetics is a multidisciplinary science about the development and self-organization of complex dynamic systems (including psychopathology development), the main functional principles of which are: non-linearity, non-stability, openness, dynamical hierarchy, observability. The methodology of synergetics is based on the integrative approach to the study of structures which are thermodynamically open, non-equilibrious, exchanging energy, information and substance with the environment of dissipative structures.

Dissipative structures are discrete self-organizing systems dissipating energy and distinguished by their spiral formation in multidimensional space, which trajectory and self-vibrating amplitude have a multivariant nature and are predetermined by a combination of differently directed forces and factors in bifurcation points. Dissipative structures exist and are formed in the society and the biosphere and intermittently go through self-organization processes following their internal development logic, becoming more complicated or degrading throughout their existence.

In synergetics, an important concept is a strange attractor. It is an object in the phase space that almost all trajectories aim for and upon which they are unstable. Attractors are classified as fractals (Latin fractus – fragmented) – objects characterized by their fractional size and multidirectionality of developmental trajectories. A fractal is a self-similar figure made up of parts that are each similar to the whole figure and have an uncommon structure. For example, fractal architecture and design are repeated at micro-, meso- and macro levels from DNA molecules to galactic spirals. In clinical medicine, a fractal is both development and state uniting time and qualitative characteristics of systems or bodies. A fractal is a projection on the scientific field of quantum concepts.

Fractal dynamics is a transition of a quantum system from one possible state to another via bifurcation, having passed which, a dissipative structure starts aiming for a new attractor. In clinical medicine, it corresponds to the development of psychosomatic disorders or recovery – depending on which of the attractors (leading to progression or remission) turns out to be currently important.

It is impossible to imagine isolated human psychosomatic health without interactions and influences of many internal and external factors. As a result, complicated and non-linear, unstable and open self-organizing dissipative systems appear.

We (Sidorov 2006, 2014) have developed a synergetic biopsycho-sociospiritual conception of ontogenesis that is represented by a tetranuclear or four-dimensional model consisting of vectors or planes of somato- and psycho-, socio- and animogenesis (Figure 1).

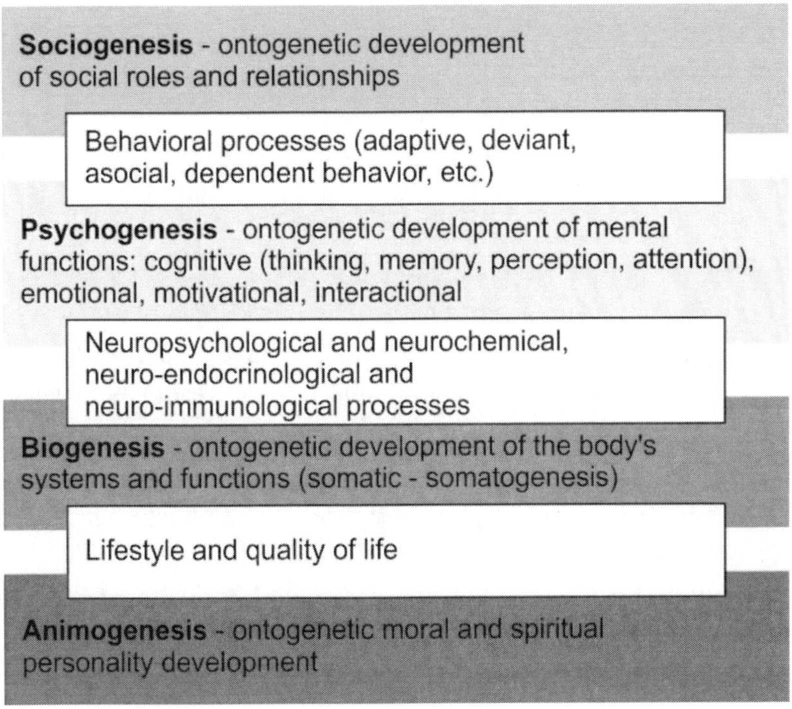

Figure 1. Biopsychosociospiritual model of ontogenesis.

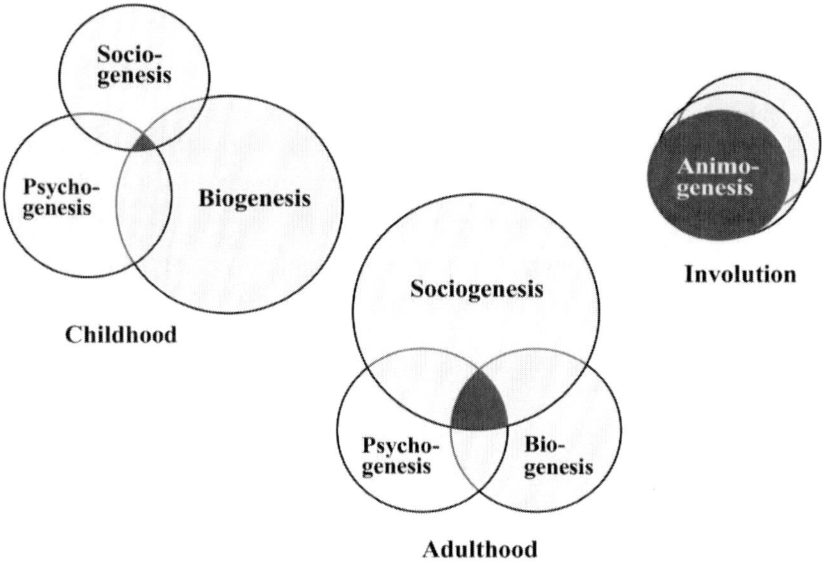

Figure 2. Dynamics of biopsychosociospiritual assimilation.

Anima, animus (Latin anima – soul, and animus – spirit) are concepts that in the Ancient Greek culture framed the phenomenon of spirit and acted as stages of the evolution of spirituality understanding: if anima (soul) is inseparable from its material carrier, then animus (spirit) has an autonomous status. Animogenesis is a term that integrates understanding of soul and spirit, specifies the central fourth part of the proposed ontogenetic model (Figure 2). The main ontogenesis planes interpenetrated and determined transit zones and a central part containing consciousness – the highest level of self-regulation and reflection of reality accumulating spiritual-moral potential.

The model presupposes a multidisciplinary and integral approach to complex and complicated psychosomatic cause-effect relationships. Trajectories of state or disease progress are determined and corrected at bifurcation points acquiring spiral-like properties and multivariance. For a better visual perception, Figure 3 presents a linear trajectory of psychosomatic diseases progress.

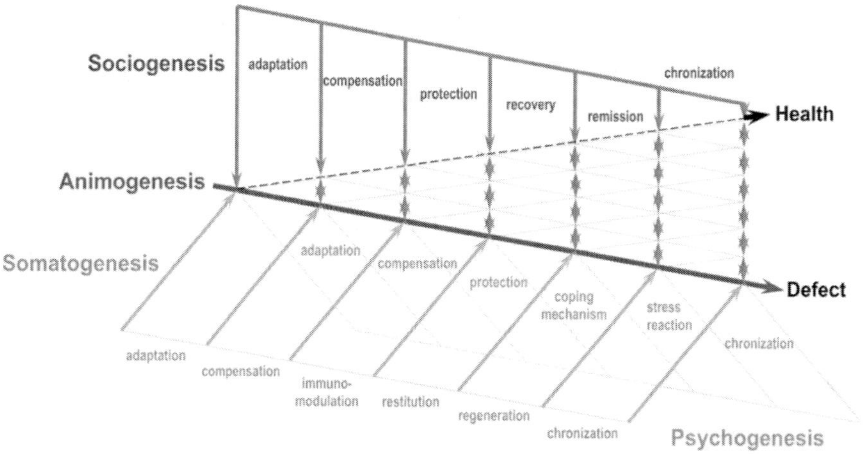

Figure 3. Fractal trajectory of states (diseases, epidemics) progress and protectional mechanisms.

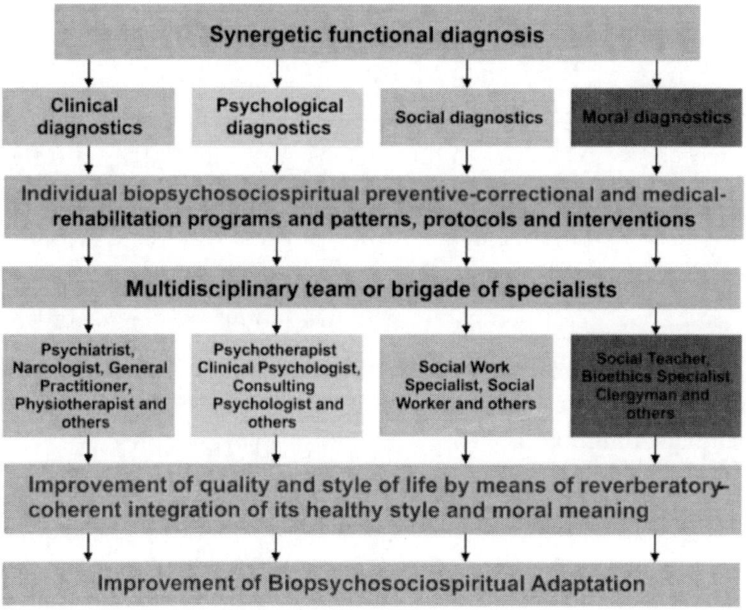

Figure 4. Synergetic functional diagnostics in mental medicine.

The traditional linear dynamics is changed by the synergetic non-linear fractality. Synergetics considers a human body as a complicated open system with non-linear processes. Such behavior is based on polymodal mechanisms of defense and appearance of internal fluctuations. After accumulation of a big number of fluctuations as risk factors echo, they produce cascade and cumulative effects at the bifurcation points changing the system development trajectory.

The proposed methodology makes it possible to formulate clinical and psychological, social and moral diagnoses taking shape of a syndromic synergetic functional diagnosis (Figure 4). Only such approach allows effectively carrying out personalized multidisciplinary protocols in mental medicine (Sidorov 2006, 2014).

2. Etiopathogenesis of the Early Psychic Trauma

Clash of the child's world with the world of adults, other children and a variety of events is not always painless for the child. Sudden life events with a high degree of probability predispose to the occurrence of child's psychic disorders. If by their nature they are psycho-traumatic, they cause the long-term adverse changes in life circumstances, lower the self-esteem.

Chronic stress, inevitable in any country in the transitional period has led to an increase in the incidence of psychogenic disorders, alcohol and drug abuse, increase in mental retardation. It is known that about 10% of all children have at least one parent who has serious psychic disorders. In recent years, there is a noticeable rise in the number of social orphans – the children, whose parents are deprived of parental rights. In Russia, there are more than half a million orphans, who are in state care, 96% of them are the orphans with living parents, who are deprived of the enshrined in the UN Convention child's right to have a family. Social stratification of the population, deterioration of living standards, weakening of the family institution has led to the increase in the number of children with the anamnesis of the early psychic trauma.

The disorder occurs more severe if the trauma is caused by human actions, rather than external factors. The most severe psychic traumas of childhood are the loss of a close adult and sexual molestation. Serious consequences are seen in the children, who suffered from the maltreatment. The emotional deprivation factors form a special group of psycho-traumatic factors (Kozlovskaya et al. 2005; Makarov 2012; Sidorov 2017).

3. Traumatogenic Syndrome of Mental Immunodeficiency

The yesterday's classic stress and then – chronic psychosocial stress, today has become an existential stress – an indispensable element of an alarming picture of the world and the way of life of almost any person. Having become so common nowadays, thousands of demonstrations on the streets of European cities with posters "We are not afraid" after each act of terrorism, are now accepted as almost a public recognition of the fact that the world is ruled by terror, which has become so familiar that people are not afraid of it anymore... That is why in mental medicine we have identified a special form of mental terrorism (MT) – destructive and explosive manipulation of consciousness. MT continues and develops the previously developed conceptual trend, described in terms of mobbing - bullying - crowding. The most dramatically MT is manifested in the psychic traumatization of childhood. An epigenetic example is the unborn children of today's migrants in the EU, experiencing complexes of refugees with their mothers, humiliated and insulted, losing self-esteem and self-respect, whose children may hate and despise yesterday's benefactors of their parents, and grandchildren are ready to blow up mentally this unbearably free world ...

Prenatal traumatic experience of modern European migrants in 3-4 generations can manifest itself literally as a "mental nuclear explosion" that destroys European identity. Romantic plans for assimilation and adaptation have long since found their inadequacy.

An important epigenetic feature of the mental weapon of the modern hybrid war is that, figuratively speaking, it aims at its target in the 1st generation, clicks on the trigger in the 2nd, the ruins of yesterday's well-being are inspected in the 3rd, and the long-term consequences become the habitual way of life for the 4th generation.

Modern chronic existential stress as a new quality of psychosocial stress through epigenetic mechanisms predetermines the activity of the genome, preparing new generations for existence in a hybrid environment – multimodal and totally socially stressful. Most of the characteristics of long-term activity of the genome are established at the stages of early development – from the prenatal period to the early maturation. It is this period that is in the focus of attention of researchers trying to explain the phenomenon of growth of psychopathology in the modern world (Vajserman et al. 2011; Rozanov 2016; Sidorov 2017).

The actual task is to describe and systemize the epigenetic dysfunctions of mental immunity, clinically manifested by the SMID and launching the epidemiological cascade: mental epidemic - destructive mental epidemic - pandemic of mental immunodeficiency.

Adverse experiences at an early age or an early life stress (ELS) have both acute and long-term effects on epigenetic labels in the brain that affect cognitive functions and behavior, the risk of suicide and psychic disorders throughout the life of present and future generations. The most studied in experimental neuroepigenetics are the mechanisms of histone modification and methylation of DNA (Griffiths, Hunter 2014). The possibility of ELS induction by epigenetic modulation of gene expression leading to altered adult phenotypes has been shown (Lewis, Olive 2014).

In the area of a long-term neuron-synaptic plasticity (Karpova et al. 2017) several regulatory mechanisms have been identified at the level of transcription and posttranscription, which include promoter activation and alternative fusion, transcript resistance and polyadenylation. New epigenetic pharmacological resources for mobilizing neural plasticity in stress disorders and neurological diseases have been revealed (Karpova et al. 2017).

A study of the neurochemical profile of adult male mice subjected to traumatic stress in the early postpartum period and their offspring found that paternal trauma can also bring beneficial effects for the brain metabolism by acute stress in offspring (Gapp et al. 2017). The perspective of neuroepigenetics of PTSD, which allows identifying and predicting new candidates for neurotherapy aimed at stressful pathogenic memories, is also shown (Blouin et al. 2016).

An experimental study of memory found an interesting clinical parallel. It turned out that the genes involved in the formation of memory in invertebrates are responsible for mental retardation in humans (Bolduc, Tully 2009).

The uniqueness of the collection of memories of a person determines personal and social identity, shaping and modeling the interaction with the world. The possibility (Sillivan et al. 2015) of developing new therapeutic goals for the treatment of PTSD and drug dependence by correcting the neuroepigenetic mechanisms of memory dysregulation is shown.

The dynamic balance between DNA methylation and demethylation of genes regulated by neuronal activity is crucial for memory processes. In a study in mice, the critical role of Tet 1 -oxidase was identified (Kumar et al. 2015) in regulating neuronal transcription and maintaining the epigenetic state of the brain associated with the memory consolidation and memory chronotope. Another study shows the role of these mechanisms in the regulation of neurophysiological spatial representation and memory formation (Roth et al. 2015). It remains an open question – how dramatic are the traces of these memories in the scale of the transgenerational models.

Emerging under stressful influence epigenetic labels fix and model the expression of gene complexes, influencing the design of the brain cell ensembles and predetermining the probability of psychic disorders (Rozanov 2016). It is interesting to note that an adverse transcriptional reaction to stress in the form of differential activation of the components of the immune system is more pronounced in people with a high hedonic component of mental health and significantly weaker in those whose psyche is based on the eudemonic well-being (Fredrickson et al. 2013).

We cannot disagree with the fact that the meaningfulness of existence and the realization of one's goals in life, spirituality and

Table 1. Clinical manifestations of MI dysfunctions in EPT

Normative function of MI	Clinic of predominant MI dysfunction
Regulatory – system resource management of MI	Decreased self-esteem and lack of self-confidence, anxiety and worry, feelings of guilt and helplessness, difficulties in differentiating perceptions of one's own and others' interests
Integrative – the unification of all types and resources of MI	Somatopsychosociospiritual lability: from vegetative-vascular dystonia and psychosomatoses, to psychotraumatic personality disorder and dyscirculatory encephalopathy
Coherent – harmonious integrity and dynamic plasticity of MI	Asthenia and rapid exhaustion, increased suggestibility and conformity, behavioral stereotyping and semantic rigidity, appetite and eating disorders
Target – actual focus and algorithmization of MI	Difficulties in building priority and sequence of activities, ease of switching and distraction, deformation and loss of protective mechanisms
Adaptive – adaptation to changing environmental conditions	The increase in isolation and alienation, hostility and aggression, a sense of hopelessness and frustration, uselessness and meaninglessness of life, systemic decompensation and demoralization, suicidal thoughts and actions
Resonance – tempo-rhythmological MI adjustment for the dynamic of challenges	Reduced synthony and altruism, fading interest in the problems of the real and virtual world, other communities and people, increasing inhibition and/or hyperactivity, depression and dysphoria (the special temperament of a difficult child)
Interactive – correction of resource design and multimodal interface of MI relative to the effectiveness of interaction	The degradation of style and way of life, the reduction and loss of alternative interests; dependent disorders and delinquency, promiscuity and prostitution (in those who have experienced sexual violence)
Mirror – accumulation of experience in mental representation	"Post-traumatic games" with obsessive memories, stereotypical nightmares and sleep disorders, psychomotor and cognitive regression with the loss of newly acquired skills, permanent anxiety and stress
Symmetric – the correspondence of the mobilized resources of MI to the variety of challenges	The increase and weighting of the abuses and delicts, psychopathy-like and somatoform disorders (by the puberty age)
Cumulative – "explosive" mobilization of MI	Verbal and motor impulsiveness, compulsiveness of attractions and actions
Prognostic – mobilization of MI, outrunning the threat	"Prognostic dullness" with ignoring the obvious consequences and complications, neglect of interaction with the family and social environment
Interiorization – the formation of new internal patterns of MI through the assimilation of external algorithms	The disharmony of the formation of psychological and social roles, moral feelings and spiritual values, a "tunnel" vision of the world and itself in it, a traumatic contusion of all forms of activity and curiosity

involvement in society (as opposed to hedonism and consumerism) create the best chances for realizing the life potential. That is why the biopsychosociospiritual methodology of MM allows the most complete approach to adaptive neuroengineering and self-management of mental health as a polymodal well-being.

Undoubtedly, attempting to bind certain epigenetic labels or switches to specific manifestations of behavioral phenomenology and clinical psychopathology may seem excessively mechanistic so far. The substantiation of the functional characteristics of MI accumulating epigenetic markers allows us isolating the predominantly disturbed function, which manifests itself in a certain pathoplasty and pathokinetics. Table 1 shows the clinical manifestations of MI dysfunction in the early trauma.

Traumatogenic SMID is represented by a variety of boundary biopsychosociospiritual identity disorders. Its pathogenetic basis consists of epigenetic accumulation of functional (reversible and dynamic) MI disorders in the "traumatogenic family". It must be admitted that today MI is in many respects a standard placeholder, denoting the missing or indefinite multidisciplinary and multimodal parameter in the network of the relationship between genome and epigenome, identity and behavior.

Studies of early childhood psychic trauma (Fredrickson et al. 2013; Sidorov 2016, 2017) have shown the multivariance of changes in MI and biopsychosociospiritual characteristics of a "traumatogenic family" depending on the severity and duration of transgenerational stress burden. Clinical scenarios and trajectories of the destinies of new generations of "traumatogenic epigenome" essentially depended on external conditions: the same behavioral models (which are always the same for humanity) gave completely opposite effects in different social environments. This requires further multidisciplinary studies of modulation of identity and behavioral navigation based on the synergetic methodology of mental medicine.

4. Synergetics of the Early Psychic Trauma

The subject of synergetics are the mechanisms of spontaneous formation and preservation of complex systems, especially in the relation to the stable disbalance with the environment (this includes all the biotic and social organisms). The focus areas of synergetics are the nonlinear effects of the evolution of the systems of all types, crises and bifurcation – unstable phases of the existence, involving a multiplicity of future scenarios for further development.

It is quite generalized and conditionally enough to present the dynamics of the early psychic trauma (EPT) from the position of the synergetic concept. Fractal dynamics is non-linear, its trajectory includes the following fractals of the biopsychosociospiritual model: predisposition, latent, initial, full-scale clinical picture, chronization and outcome (Table 2).

Feelings traumas, associated with the loss of the object of love, at first sight, seem unexpected. A study of family situations, in which the child suffered a psychic trauma, demonstrates the advanced readiness to the psychic trauma process. Here *the predisposition fractal – family dysontogenesis of the traumatogenic family* – begins. Unstable relationships, high level of emotional expression, lack of support, proneness to conflict, and hostility are the characteristic features of this family, identified with the help of projective techniques among children, who had the trauma. Lack of family traditions and spiritual values, addiction and affective disorders were observed among the parents. Low morale, educational and material levels are typical. Child-rearing is held according to the type of emotional rejection and hypo-care, which entails the development of emotional and spiritual-moral deficit. Disharmony in family relationships predisposes to a distortion of moral socialization process of the child in the future.

Unfavorable hereditary burden under the influence of unfavorable factors of the environment triggers psycho-vegetative imbalance.

The following is a *latent fractal of pre-traumatic diathesis* (psychic diathesis is a set of features, which characterizes the predisposition to psychic pathology). In most cases, it is represented by a special temperament of the "problem child" – a very movable, in a bad mood, hardly adaptable. It is known that the more acute and massive is the psychic trauma, the lesser role is played by personal characteristics of the child. With a decrease in the severity and the intensity of the trauma, the individual characteristics become major in the formation of the clinical picture of the post-traumatic period (Zakharov 1988). This is especially true for the compulsive and asthenia traits. The younger is the child, the more severe are the somatic-vegetative symptoms.

Violation of neural processes is shown through the disharmony of moral feelings formation, which in future can predetermine the violation of moral socialization and development of the personality, which has low adaptive potential.

This is followed by an *initial fractal of functional disorders* – the actual psychic trauma. Children are more sensitive to the trauma. The younger is the child, the more dramatically the event is perceived, as the ability to assimilate and integrate the trauma in the childhood experiences is lower. After trauma, children frequently repeat the psycho-traumatic situation in games ("post-traumatic games"); there are nightmares, increased confusion, avoidance of social contacts, psychomotor regression with loss of recently learned skills, sleep disorder, the emergence of various fears (Korneyev 1996). This is accompanied by excessive excitability of the autonomic nervous system, high levels of wakefulness. There is a transient social dysfunction.

Vegetative-vascular dystonia and neurotic reactions are shown through the multi-variant deformation of the moral character, laying the foundation for the future development of the demoralization syndrome.

This is followed by a fractal of a full-scale clinical picture, when there are the comorbid disorders on the background of the traumatic stress disorder. Children's behavior resembles a picture of psychopathic state. But the similarity is only superficial, because the traumatized children experience depression, anxiety, feeling of guilt, uselessness of life, suicidal thoughts.

Table 2. Fractal dynamics of the epidemic development of the early psychic trauma

Ontogenesis vector	Prenosological fractals			Nosological fractals		
	Predisposition: traumatogenic family	**Latent:** pre-traumatic diathesis	**Initial:** functional disorders	**Full-scale clinical picture**/mental epidemic	**Chronization:** forms and types of the course/destructive mental epidemic	**Outcome/** pandemic
Somatogenesis	Hereditary burden	Violation of neuro-processes	Vegetative-vascular abnormalities	Somatoform vegetative disfunction	Somatoform disorders	Dyscirculatory encephalopathy
Psychogenesis	Family with an increased willingness to a psychic trauma	Compulsive and asthenic traits of the "difficult teenager"	Psychomotor regression, fears and nightmares, confusion	Post-traumatic stress disorder	Post-reactive formation of personality	Personality disorder
Sociogenesis	Disharmonious family relationships	Violation of socialization	Transient social dysfunction	Violation of social ties	Social decompensation	Social deadaptation
Animogenesis	Spiritual-moral deficiency or ambivalence of the family	Disharmony of moral sentiments formation	Violations of moral character	Loss of spiritual and moral position	Probability of immoral acts	Probability of illegal behavior

Somatic complaints increase, psychosomatic pathology is formed.

Neuroanatomical effects are shown through the decrease in volume of the hippocampus, expressed by the dextrocerebral asymmetry, decreased activity of the Broca area during the "flash-back" (perhaps, this explains why it is particularly difficult to give words to their experiences for children with PTSD (Jacobson, Jacobson 2006).

Social ties are breaking, which is caused by the increasing hostility towards the world around and the lack of interest to other people's problems.

The memory of the past is always present, but it can influence the course of life just before the bifurcation points, i.e., the decisive moments of selecting one of the possible ways of life. If the bifurcation point is passed, the path selection is done, and then the activity is determined by one of the structures of development attractors. If the traumatic past dominates over the future, and the future becomes not obvious, the fate of the trajectory is distorted.

Since the psychological past, present and future are the parts of the psychological field, both the past (past experience), and the future (expectations, desires, fears and dreams) affect the forces, which govern the individual behavior today. Psychic trauma violates this balance towards the past, creating a hostile, skeptical attitude towards the world, social estrangement, hopelessness, chronic feeling of anxiety, alienation.

Animogenesis of the somatoform dysfunction is shown through the destruction of spiritual-moral position of the child, embodied in the early development of the demoralization syndrome.

The situation is changed by the synchronized oscillations near the bifurcation point; a close adult, located nearby, who creates an atmosphere of security, changes the future. If this is not feasible, there is the *chronization fractal* – the postreactive personality formation, which occurs on the basis of a prolonged neurosis and is characterized by a combination of dynamic pathological changes in the character and fixed neurotic disorders. The clinical picture of this period is characterized by a combination of psychopathic-like and severe neurosis-like disorders.

Emotional disturbances of this EPT fractal are strongly colored with the somatic symptoms, which often come to the fore in the form of somatoform disorders.

In social terms, the adaptation deterioration leads to the social decompensation, and there is a risk of immoral acts in the animogenesis.

Final EPT fractal is the *fractal of outcome*, a personality disorder. Psychotraumatic personality disorder is formed, as a rule, not earlier than puberty age. A wide range of behavioral problems comes to the foreground. Various offences, dependence on psychoactive substances, suicidal thoughts are typical. Sexually abused girls often become prostitutes.

Somatoneurological complications of this period consist of sleep disorders, loss of appetite, eating disorders, amplification of somatoneurological complaints, the development of vascular encephalopathy. Social disadaptation with a high risk of asocial personality development takes place at this stage.

Psychic traumas, experienced in childhood, form the adult destiny, which is not a priori dramatic. Traditionally, the severity of trauma and its damaging action are determined by the intensity of exposure without taking into account the surrounding circumstances. We studied the research of children of latent age, who underwent the psychic trauma in past medical history (feelings traumas, related to the loss of the love object – the death of parents, abusive treatment, sexual abuse, social orphanhood). Identified deviations of the studied parameters (intelligence, personality characteristics, "self-concept", bioelectrical activity of brain and the artistic creativity of children) with the same nature of the trauma forced us to turn to a favorite image of the synergetics – the bifurcation model.

In the bifurcation points there is the selection of the path; the processes of another level (accidents) in the vicinity of bifurcation points can play a key role. Here such "accidents" are the circumstances related to the trauma – absence of close adult nearby, the situation of disregard, humiliation and bad care, age of the early psychic trauma till 7 years, the existence of special temperament among "problem children", being in the orphanage, absence of professional assistance. The mechanisms, at the expense of which the psychic trauma causes psychic disorders in the remote period, include mainly the presence or absence of a close adult nearby. Close adult and traumatized child must enter into a relationship of social attraction, based on the sustainable positive feelings to each other. This means that the path of development of post-traumatic period is not the only one. If we find the right moment to intervene in the course of events, it is possible to change it.

5. Method for Determining the EPT Severity Degree

We have developed a method for determining the severity of the EPT, which focuses on the accidents of near bifurcation points. Namely they determine the result of the post-traumatic period.

The algorithm of actions consists of two consecutive blocks. In the first (I) block, the nature of psychic trauma is evaluated: the short-term psychic trauma (STPT), factors of emotional deprivation (FED), chronic psychic trauma (CPT). STPT occurs among children, whose parents died as a result of a family conflict, suicide or illness (STPT-1), or which are the victims of sexual violence (STPT-2). These EPT are ranked by us with the maximum number of points - 50 and 30 points respectively (see Table 3).

The second group, according to the EPT severity, is FED-1 (social orphans, including the children, abandoned by their parents in the hospital, having no relationship with biological parents).

CPT group (child abuse) is estimated by us in 20 points. FED-2 group (social orphans, having relationships with biological parents, and the children, adopted at the age of 4–7 years) – in 10 points.

Block II includes a list of desynchronizing fluctuations (aggravating circumstances): the lack of trusting relationship with someone in the immediate surround, the situation of disregard, poor care and humiliation, the age of trauma before seven years. The presence of a special type of temperament – “problem child” (full of play, is in a bad mood, is difficult to adapt), being in an orphan house, the lack of professional help, low economic status of the family, who are ranked on a scale from 1 to 7.

Table 3. Assessment of the early psychic trauma severity, points

Points	**Block I: the nature of psychic trauma**
50	STPT-1 Children, whose parents died (as a result of family conflict, suicide or illness)
40	FED-1 Social orphans (children, who were abandoned in the hospital), not maintaining relations with parents
30	STPT-2 Children – victims of sexual violence
20	CPT Children, suffered from abusive treatment
10	FED-2 Social orphans, having relationships with biological parents, and the children, adopted at the age of 4-7 years
Block II: aggravating circumstances	
7	Lack of a trusting relationship with anyone in the immediate surround
6	Situation of disregard, poor care and humiliation
5	Age till 7 years
4	Presence of a special type of temperament – “problem child”
3	Being in the orphanage
2	Absence of professional assistance (psychologists and psychiatrists)
1	Low economic status
	Total number of points

In order to determine the severity of the EPT, it is necessary to put a mark in the block 1, according to the nature of the EPT. Each case can be attributed to only one category of trauma.

Then it is necessary to evaluate the aggravating circumstances. Several aggravating circumstances can be added together, then the points of blocks I and II are added. Minimum number of points – 13, maximum – 78. EPT are divided into three groups of severity: trauma, estimated in 13-34 points, refers to mild degree; 35-56 points - to moderate; 57-78 points - to severe.

Example No. 1: The Child A.

8 years, the patient of the Children department of the Arkhangelsk Regional Clinical Psychiatric Hospital (ARCPH), dealt with complaints of auto-aggressive behavior, anxiety, disturbed sleep, inability to maintain a friendly relationship with children, restlessness, excessive mobility, aggressiveness and poor school performance.

At the age of 4, the boy suffered the early psychic trauma: in his presence, his mother, being in a state of pathological alcohol intoxication, killed his father, grandmother, grandfather and younger brother; he survived by a miracle. After the arrest of his mother, he was placed in the orphanage. Professional assistance was not provided. He was perceived by others as mentally retarded. He was afraid of adults and children. Nearby there was no adult, who would be able to create close trust-based relations. In addition, the poor child care in the child's home was a common thing; the other kids bullied the boy.

Assessment of the severity of the EPT was carried out with taking into account the nature of the psychic trauma and aggravating circumstances:

Block I (EPT nature) – STPT-1 (parents died as a result of family conflict) – 50 points;

Block II:

1. lack of trusting relationship with anyone in the immediate surrounding – 7 points;
2. situation of disregard, poor care and humiliation – 6 points;
3. age of EPT before 7 years – 5 points;
4. presence of a particular temperament "problem child" – 4 points;
5. being in the orphanage – 3 points;
6. absence of professional assistance – 2 points.

Total score = block I points + block II points = 50 + 27 = 77 points, which corresponds to severe EPT.

Example No. 2: Patient N

11 years, was admitted to the Children department of the ARCPH with complaints of verbal aggression toward adults, escapes from the children's home, easy crying.
Born in prison, where she was living with her mother for 3 years, then taken to the orphanage. There she was calm, docile, friendly. She developed a close positive relationship with one of the teachers. The atmosphere in the child's home was warm. Two years ago her mother was released from prison, she settled down not far from the girl, supported a relationship with her, even though they did not quite satisfy the child.

Calculation of the EPT severity:

1. nature of the EPT – FED (social orphans, having supportive relationships with biological parents) – 10 points;
2. age of EPT before 7 years – 5 points;
3. being in the orphanage – 3 points;
4. absence of professional assistance – 2 points.

According to the table of the EPT evaluation, the patient collects 20 points, which corresponds to the mild severity level.

6. Medico-Psychosociospiritual Care

To prevent severe consequences of an early psychic trauma, we (Sidorov, Yakovleva 2014) developed a program of medico-psychosociospiritual assistance to children, which is based on the concept of synergetics. The program consists of four blocks (see Table 4): medical and psychological, social and spiritual-moral, involving the multidisciplinary teams to assist with the participation of pediatricians, pediatric neurologists and psychiatrists, psychologists, psychotherapists, social workers and teachers. Preventive measures need to begin even in the *predisposition fractal*; they are aimed at improving the environment, in which a child is brought up, ethical psychological harmonization of the parents individuality and family relations.

The *latent fractal* focuses on the identification of the predisposition to psychic disorders, on the diathesis diagnostics, increased stress resistance and harmonization of moral socialization of the personality.

In the *initial fractal*, the diagnostics of traumatic disorders becomes the most important, since in many cases they remain unrecognized and the provision of timely qualified assistance is impossible. Creating the security situation, supportive, trusting relationships with close adults, good care and professional help at this stage can reduce the negative effects, preventing the neurotic disorders among children and correcting the formation of their moral character.

In the fractal of a *full-scale clinical picture*, when the comorbid disorders start to appear, it is important to promote the integration of the traumatic experience into the events of the current child life; to foster the adaption to the new situation; to carry out the medicated and psychotherapeutic social and spiritual-moral correction.

The fractal of the process of chronization dictates the emphasis on the fight against social and moral exclusion with the help of psychotherapeutic and pedagogic strategies.

Fractal of the PTSD outcome – personality disorder – requires medical and psychological, social and spiritual moral rehabilitation.

Thus, the dynamics of the early psychic trauma includes the following fractals: predisposition – special traumatogenic family with increased willingness to psychic traumatization of children, being brought up in it; latent – pretraumatic diathesis; initial – traumatic stress disorder, full-scale clinical picture – neurotic and affective disorders; chronization – postreactive formation of the person; the outcome – personality disorder.

Table 4. Medico-psychosociospiritual care program for early psychic trauma

Blocks	**Prenosological fractals**			**Nosological fractals**		
	Predisposition: traumatogenic family	**Latent:** pre-traumatic diathesis	**Initial:** functional disorders	**Full-scale clinical picture**/mental epidemic	**Chronization**: forms and types of the course/destructive mental epidemic	**Outcome**/pandemic
Spiritual and moral	Screening and correction of “morale climate” of the family	Correction of the formation and development of moral sentiments	Correction of the formation and development of moral character	Reconstruction of a moral position	Reconstruction of moral behavior	Spiritual and moral rehabilitation
Medical	Improvement of the family in which a child is brought up	Identification of individuals with different diatheses, disorders correction	Timely diagnostics of traumatic disorders	Medicated (SSRIs) and psychotherapeutic correction	Group, behavioral, individual psychotherapy	Adequate medication therapy and psychotherapy
Psychological	Identification of individuals (parents) with personality disorders, its correction	Increase of stress resistance	Creating the security situation and the possibility of semantic processing of trauma	Integration of the traumatic experience in the current life events	Psycho-pedagogical correction	Psychological rehabilitation
Social	Identification and correction of family relationships	Harmonisation of the personality socialization	Support, trusting relationships with close adults, good care	Adaptation to the situation	Fight against social exclusion	Social rehabilitation

A family with an increased willingness to psychic traumatization of children differs by the unstable relationships, lack of support from family members to each other and traditions, proneness to conflict, hostility, addiction of parents, low moral, educational and material level. Pretraumatic diathesis is a borderline state, which under the influence of exogenous factors is transformed into the illness. Presence of the "problem child" temperament worsens the PTSD course. An initial period of the EPT is the actual traumatic stress disorder.

Accompanying circumstances will determine the PTSD course. Lack of close trust relations, poor care, humiliation, the age before seven years, the lack of professional assistance, staying in the orphanage – worsen the prognosis. The full-scale clinical picture includes the neurotic and affective disorders, hiding under the guise of psychopathic-like symptoms. Postreactive personality formation in the absence of favorable attendant circumstances is completed with the personality disorder.

The medico-psychosociospiritual care program for early psychic trauma, developed on the basis of the synergetic concept, includes the medical and psychological, spiritual-moral and social blocks, and involves the multidisciplinary teams in the prevention, correction and rehabilitation.

Synergetic methodology takes into account all the internal and external factors of an early psychic trauma and allows preventing its dire consequences, stopping the generalization of mental epidemic.

CONCLUSION

The geometric growth in the number of publications on neuroepigenetics and the rapid evolution of its research field actualize the definition of epistemological and philosophical-gnoseological boundaries, as well as the instrumental and technological opportunities of multidisciplinary interaction for obtaining practically meaningful clinical results. MM is one of the newest examples of reformatting yesterday's nosocentric boundaries and early pre-nosological forecasting of tomorrow's possible mental ailments. The multidisciplinary synergetic biopsychosociospiritual methodology of MM is in demand in new discourses of neuroepigenetics according to the mechanisms of the influence of the environment on the brain and behavior. The substantiation for the functional lateralization of mentality (mental asymmetry) as one of the tools of neuroepigenetic coding of identity and behavior is proposed. MM harmoniously combines in its technological platform genetic and epigenetic molecular mechanisms, socio-psychological and clinical-psychopathological, spiritual-moral and religious-integrated tools. This allows MM to practically implement yesterday's "neuroepigenetic fantasies" about editing and formatting the design of the network cascade of genetic and epigenetic identity: molecular - cellular - tissue - organ - organism - personal - social - population. The degree and the vector of dispersion of genomic and epigenomic identity reflect possible resources of evolutionary variability embodied in the registers of MI and manifested by the mental resilience. MI is a neural network multisystem and multimodal identity and consciousness interface in its interaction with the internal and external environment. The identified 12 basic functional characteristics of MI are modeled by epigenetic switches or labels, and are embodied in behavioral phenomenology or pathoplasty and pathokinetics of mental disorders. The epidemic increase in the prevalence of mental and psychosomatic disorders is suggested to be called the PMID by the name of the earliest and nonspecific syndrome of mental immunodeficiency accumulating initial manifestations of MI dysfunctions transgenerationally. The global predictors of PMID are many of the challenges of the modern world: from the psychic traumatization of childhood to cumulative existential stress. The biological core of MI is the hypothalamic-pituitary-adrenal axis, which provides epigenetic stress-modulation together with stress-sensitive areas of the brain. In MM, sanogenetic therapy as adaptive modulation of MI triggers cascade self-renewal of personality, clinically manifested by its therapeutic drift (diagnoses-syndromes-symptoms-states). The well-known expression of Nobel Laureate Peter Medawar: "*Genetics* proposes and *epigenetics* disposes" should be supplemented with a practically significant mission of MM, which embodies the design models of quality and style, the way and meaning of life in adaptive neuroengineering and self-management of consciousness and health.

References

Blouin, A. M., Sillivan, S. E., Joseph, N. F., Miller, C. A. (2016). The potential of epigenetics in stress-enhanced fear learning models of PTSD // *Learn Mem*. 23 (10), pp. 576-586.

Bolduc, F. V., Tully, T. (2009). Fruit flies and intellectual disability // *Fly (Austin)*. V.3. № 1. pp. 91-104.

Fredrickson, B. L. et al. (2013). A functional genomic perspective on human well-being // *PNAS*. V. 110. № 33. P. 13684-9.

Gapp, K., Corcoba, A., van Steenwyk, G., Mansuy, I. M., Duarte, J. M. (2017). Brain metabolic alterations in mice subjected to postnatal traumatic stress and in their offspring // *J Cereb Blood Flow Metab*. V. 37 (7), pp. 2423-2432.

Griffiths, B. B., Hunter, R. G. (2014). Neuroepigenetics of stress // *Neuroscience*. V. 275, pp. 420-435.

Jacobson, J. L., Jacobson, A. M. (2006). *Psychiatric Secrets*. London. Elsevier. P. 576.

Karpova, N. N., Sales, A. J., Joca, S. R. (2017). Epigenetic Basis of Neuronal and Synaptic Plasticity // *Current Topics In Medicinal Chemistry*. V. 17 (7). pp. 771-793.

Korneyev, A. S. (1996). O klassifikatsii psikhicheskikh rasstroistv u detei rannego vozrasta// *Sbornik nauchnykh trudov Sankt-Peterburgskogo instituta rannego vmeshatel'stva.* [On the classification of mental disorders in young children // *Collection of proceedings of the St. Petersburg Institute of Early Intervention*]. V. 1. pp. 41-44. [in Russian].

Kozlovskaya, G. V., Proselkova, M. E., Kalinina, M. A., Margolina, I. A., Platonova, N. V. (2005). Psihicheskaya deprivatsiya kak patogennyiy faktor v rannem ontogeneze // *Psihiatriya*. [Psychic deprivation as a pathogene at the early stage of early ontogenesis // *Psychiatry*]. 6, pp. 18-23. [in Russian].

Kumar, D., Aggarwal, M., Kaas, G. A. et al. (2015). Tet1 Oxidase Regulates Neuronal Gene Transcription, Active DNA Hydroxy-methylation, Object Location Memory, and Threat Recognition Memory // *Neuroepigenetics*. V. 4, pp. 12-27.

Lewis, C. R., Olive, M. F. (2014). Early-life stress interactions with the epigenome: potential mechanisms driving vulnerability toward psychiatric illness // *Behav Pharmacol*. V. 25 (5-6), pp. 341-51.

Makarov, V. V., Makarov, G. A. (2012). *Ekspedicii dushi: psihoterapija, duhovnost* [*Expeditions of the soul: psychotherapy and spirituality*]. M.: Academic Project, P. 305. [in Russian].

Roth, E. D., Roth, T. L., Money, K. M. et al. (2015). DNA methylation regulates neurophysiological spatial representation in memory formation // *Neuroepigenetics*. V. 2, pp. 1-8.

Rozanov, V. A. (2016). Psihosocial'nyj stress, epigenetika i programmirovanie psihicheskogo zdorov'ya // *Psihicheskoe zdorov'e cheloveka XXI veka*. [Psychosocial stress, epigenetics and programming of mental health // *Mental health of the XXI century*]: Collection of scientific articles on the materials of the Congress. M.: Gorodec. pp. 273-276. [in Russian].

Sidorov, P. I. (2006). *Narkologicheskaya preventologiya. Rukovodstvo. 2-e izd.* [Narcological Preventology. Handbook]. M.: MEDpress-inform. P. 720. [in Russian].

Sidorov, P. I. (2014). From bullying to pandemy of terrorism: synergetic bio-psycho-socio-spiritual methodology of mental health protection. *Handbook on Bullying: Prevalence, Psychological impacts and intervention Strategies*. NY, NOVA Science Publishers, pp. 177-214.

Sidorov, P. I. (2016). *Mental epidemics: from mobbing to terrorism*. - NY: Nova Science Publishers. P 498.

Sidorov, P. I. (2017). *Mental'naya medicina: adaptivnoe upravlenie soznaniem i zdorov'em. Rukovodstvo.* [*Mental Medicine: Adaptive Control of Mind and Health. Handbook*]. 4th ed. M.: GEOTAR-Media. P. 736. [in Russian].

Sidorov, P. I., Yakovleva, V. P. (2014). Mentalnaya ekologiya ranney psihicheskoy travmy // *Ekologiya cheloveka.* [Mental Ecology of the Early Psychic Trauma // *Human Ecology*]. V. 9. pp. 35-41. [in Russian].

Sillivan, S. E., Vaissière, T., Miller, C. A. (2015). Neuroepigenetic Regulation of Pathogenic Memories // *Neuroepigenetics*. V. 1, pp. 28-33.

Vajserman, A. M., Vojtenko, V. P., Mekhova, L. V. (2011). Epigeneticheskaya epidemiologiya vozrast – zavisimyh zabolevanij // *Ontogenez* [Epigenetic Epidemiology – the Age of Dependent Disorders // *Ontogenesis*]. V. 42. №1. pp. 30-50. [in Russian].

Zakharov, A. I. (1988). *Nevrozy u detei i podrostkov [Neuroses among children and teenagers].* Moscow, Meditsina Publ. P. 248. [in Russian].

About the Editor

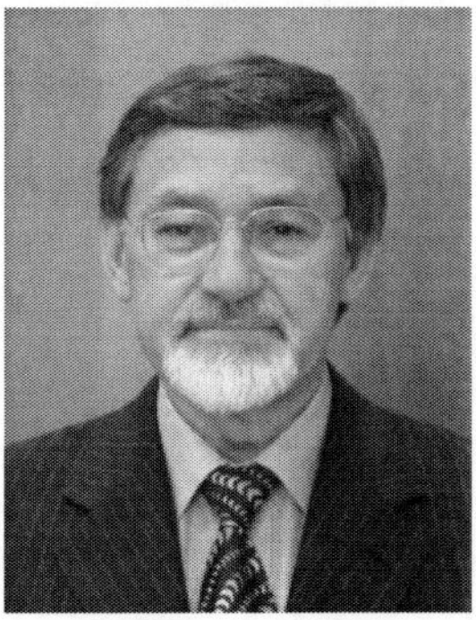

Pavel I. Sidorov, MD, PhD

Education

Arkhangelsk State Medical Institute, Medical Faculty (1976).

The All-Russian State Distance-Learning Institute of Finance and Economics, Management (2000).

Degrees and titles

Doctor of Medical Sciences, Professor, Academician of the Russian Academy of Sciences.

Candidate's dissertation on "Clinical-Social Aspects of Alcoholization and Alcoholism in Teens and Adolescents" (1979)".

Doctoral thesis on "Pathogenesis of Alcoholism in Teens and Early Prevention Methods in the Northern European Environment" (1986).

Academic Career

In 1980, began to work as an assistant in the Psychiatry department, of which he was made a professor in 1988, and in 1994, was the head of the department (until 2012).

In 1991, was made Prorector of scientific work and in 1993, became rector of ASMI.

In 1994, changed the institution into an academy and in 2000, changed it into Northern State Medical University.

At NSMU, Pavel Ivanovich opened twelve institutes, two research institutes for maritime medicine and arctic medicine, 18 specialties, nine areas of study for bachelor's degrees, and three international master's degree programs. This paved the way for the NSMU's multidisciplinary science, educational and practical innovation complex for integrated medicine based on a synergetic biology, psychology, sociology and spiritual technological platform. In 1992, the institution's economic development driver was Medipark (the medical analog of a technology park), uniting dozens of venture capital companies of varying forms of ownership and working under a public-private sector partnership (which was only legitimized in August 2009).

In 1991, he opened the first doctoral dissertation council in Russia for new specialists of emergency safety, and it was the only one of its kind in the country for six years. Under the guidance of the Russian Academy of Medical Sciences, in 1994, he launched the Human Ecology, a monthly practical science journal, and Narcology in 2002. He was the first Russian scientist admitted into the RAMS under the new specialty of human ecology; in 1995, he became a Corresponding Member and in 2000, he became an Academician.

He developed and implemented a synergetic methodology for system monitoring in a number of pilot programs, ranging from the ecological to the educational and from public health to public conscience. In 2007, after years of medical and ecological research into issues of safety at the

Plesetsk Cosmodrome, Pavel Sidorov and his colleagues published a monograph on "System Monitoring of Rocket and Space Activity" (MEDpress-inform), which warned Roscosmos leadership of the increasing probability of catastrophe in the field due to the cumulative buildup of the effects of ineffective post-Soviet models of production and management.

In 2009, Pavel Ivanovich opened the Institute of Mental Medicine in NSMU and in 2011, the Social Faculty of Mental Health was opened in a new kind of partnership with both public and private sectors and with the Russian Orthodox Church and business community. The field of "mental medicine", developed by P.I. Sidorov as a psychiatric paradigm for personalized and prognostic integrated medicine, allows for the mobilization of new interdisciplinary resources in the adaptive management of mind and health. Today, it is one of the priorities of the presidential initiatives: "Strategies for the Development of Nanoindustry" and "Strategies for Scientific and Technological Development of Russia" set to develop over the next ten to twenty years.

P.I. Sidorov has been an advisor for the defense of 38 doctoral and 45 candidate's dissertations. He is the founder of mental ecology and medicine, mental epidemiology and preventology, the conception of the system monitoring of mental health and synergetic technological platform for mental health services.

Academician P.I. Sidorov is a recognized leader in human ecology and social psychiatry, clinical psychology and disaster medicine, social epidemiology and conflictology as well as the prevention of extremism and terrorism.

Criminal Proceedings

In April 2009, in an interview with the newspaper "Pravda Severa", Pavel Sidorov spoke sharply against the transmission of NSMU into the structure of the newly created high school. The next day he was arrested while "taking bribes" from his patient and debtor, who appeared to be a drug dealer. He spent seven months in prison in Arkhangelsk. On own experience he has denied the illusion of Elbert G. Hubbard, that "prison - is a socialist paradise, where there is equality and the needs are met ..." After the death in prison "Sailor's Silence" of S. Magnitsky in November 2009, in a comatose state he was transported to the emergency department of the city hospital. In the court proceedings he submitted numerous documents of researchers receiving salaries in the "Medipark" for a total amount substantially greater than the prosecution figure. He did not admit "guilt" and was sentenced conditionally. Since 2012 he works as a chief scientific officer in NSMU. Over the years of condemnation, every month Pavel Sidorov wrote and published scientific articles, which have become the chapters of "Mental medicine". On his own experience he has shown the effectiveness of sanogenetic therapy in conditions of modern "sharashkas" (shady business establishment – *translator's note*) that have evolved significantly since the Stalin era of the Solzhenitsyn's "first round". A conditional sentence was vacated, and a criminal record was expunged in 2016. In the history of psychiatry, he was the only psychiatrist jailed by his own patient. This is the newest clinical example of the "normative anomie" and inversion of the "abuse of psychiatry" in the spectaclised world.

Honorary Titles, Awards and Prizes

In 1992, the Russian Association of Narcologists named Pavel Sidorov The Narcologist of the Year. Also he has been given the following honors: Distinguished Scientist of the RF (1997); Government of the RF Award for Science and Technology (2006) for the work on ecological system monitoring as a national security priority; 6 State Medals of the RF; Golden Badge of Honor of the Social Conscience National Foundation; Golden Psyche Psychological Competition Winner; Lomonosov Foundation Regional Prize (for creating as a native of the Kholmogorsky Region the Association of Descendents of Lomonosov). Pavel Ivanovish was awarded the Patriarch of Moscow and Russia Alexei II Certificate of Honor; the Albert Schweitzer Gold Medal; and the Polish Academy of Medicine Award for the Healthcare Service. In 2009, the World Federation of Circumpolar Medicine awarded him the Jack Hildes Medal for outstanding contribution to the development of new synergetic paradigms in arctic medicine as a hybrid system of health safety in extreme environments.

Academic Interests

Methodology of mental ecology and medicine, mental epidemiology and preventology, social psychiatry and narcology, clinical psychiatry and disaster medicine.

Academician P.I. Sidorov has made a fundamental contribution to the understanding and development of preventative systems for mental and social epidemics; the creation of original synergetic biopsycho-sociospiritual methodologies for evaluating and forecasting ontogenetic development; justifications for including terrorism and extremism within the group of polymodal and polymorphic related disorders; the conception of mental terrorism (commercial manipulation of conscience by means of threats, sanctions, etc.) as a nonlethal weapon of mass destruction; the creation of sanogenetic therapy – adaptation of the biopsychosociospiritual management of conscience and health (a priority since 1988); the validation of animogenetic (spiritual-moral) diagnostic and propaedeutic therapy and rehabilitation; the development of a multidisciplinary ideology and synergetic methodology of the mental health care and system monitoring as a social conscience interface.

Scientific Publications

Pavel Sidorov is the author of over 500 works, including 56 books and monographs, 30 textbooks and manuals, 400 journal articles (120 published in foreign journals), and 31 invention patents.

Several of his books have won awards and prizes:

a) Psychology, Clinics, and Early Prevention of Alcoholism (1984, coauthor B.S. Bratus) – the RSFSR gold medal winner of the Republican Competition of Scientific Works. The book was dedicated to his teacher, Professor I.D. Muratova, who helped open the first teen narcology office in the USSR in 1974;
b) System Monitoring of Educational Environments (2007, coauthor E.Y. Vasilyeva) – best scientific work according to the All-Russia Competition Foundation for the Development of Domestic Education.

c) Personnel Management (2008, coauthor V.I. Starodubov and I.A. Konopleva), Narcological Preventology (2008) – winners in several thematic categories of the 2008 University Book competition;
d) Perinatal Psychology and Psychiatry (2009, coauthor N.N. Volodin, et al.) – winner of the all-Russia (VDNKh) and international (Paris) book exhibitions for academic literature for innovative education (2015).

Academician P.I. Sidorov has published the next generation of federal textbooks on clinical psychology (five publications), disaster psychology and disaster medicine (four publications), perinatal psychiatry (two publications) and medico-social work (three publications), personnel management and organization (two publications), addictological preventology (four publications) and social psychiatry (two publications), human ecology (two publications) and maritime medicine (four publications), business communication (four publications) and system monitoring of educational environments (two publications), physiological foundations of human health (three publications) and psychosomatic medicine (two publications), adaptive professiogenesis (two publications) and medical law (three publications), all of which are written using a synergetic methodology of integrated medicine.

Academician P.I. Sidorov is the editor of a number of Russian translations of works on psychiatry and psychotherapy, psychology and disaster medicine from English, German, Swedish, Finnish, Norwegian, and Polish. He is a member of editorial boards of 15 all-Russian and international scientific journals.

Over the last 20 years, he has developed a synergetic biopsycho-sociospiritual methodology of mental medicine which effectively provides an adaptive management of mind and health. He has taken part in the publication of a number of handbooks employing this methodology:

1. Sidorov, P. I. (1995). *Russian Alcohol Culture. International Handbook on Alcohol and Culture*. Greenwood Press: Westport, Connecticut, London. pp. 237-253.

2. Sidorov, P. I. (2006). *Narkologicheskaya preventologiya [Narcological Preventology]*. Rukovodstvo. 2-e izd. M.: MEDpress-inform. P. 720 [in Russian].
3. Sidorov, P. I. (2014). From Bullying to Pandemy of Terrorism: Synergetic Biopsychosociospiritual Methodology of Mental Health Protection. *Handbook on Bullying: Prevalence, Psychological impacts and intervention Strategies.* NY: NOVA Science Publishers, pp. 177-214.
4. Sidorov, P. I. (2015). Mental Terrorism of Hybrid Wars and Defense Synergetics. *Handbook on New Developments in Surveillance Systems and National Security*. NY: NOVA Science Publishers. pp. 92-136.
5. Sidorov, P. I. (2015). From Mental Epidemics to Terrorism Pandemic: Synergetic Biopsychosociospiritual Methodology of Public Conscience Protection. *Handbook on Terrorism.* NY: NOVA Science Publishers. pp. 115-158.
6. Sidorov, P. I. (2016). *Mental Epidemics: From Mobbing to Terrorism. Handbook.* NY: NOVA Science Publishers. P. 498.
7. Sidorov, P. I. (2017). Epidemics of Mental Immunodeficiency as a Predictor of the Civil War. *Handbook on Civil Wars: Causal Factors, Conflict Resolution and Global Consequences.* Global Political Studies. NY: NOVA Science Publishers. pp. 55-87.
8. Sidorov, P. I. (2017). *Mentalnaya Medicina. Adaptivnoye Upravleniye Soznaniyem i Zdorovyem. Rukovodstvo. [Mental Medicine. Adaptive Management of Mind and Health. Handbook].* Moscow: Geotar-media. P. 736. [in Russian].

INDEX

A

D

E

F

N

Q

R

S